A
SOLITARY
CONFINEMENT

Robin Sheppard

Ecademy Press
6 Woodland Rise, Penryn, Cornwall TR10 8QD, UK
info@ecademy-press.com • www.ecademy-press.com

ISBN: 978-1-905823-25-3

First published 2007 by Ecademy Press

Printed and Bound by:
Lightning Source in the UK and USA

Printed on acid-free paper from managed forests. This book is printed on demand, so no copies will be remaindered or pulped.

A CIP catalogue record for this book is available from the British Library.

About the Author

Robin Sheppard had always seemed like a lucky guy! Proud father of two sons in their late teens, Sam the eldest (the musical one) and Charlie (the artistic one); still good friends with his first wife Georgina known always as George and partnered by the effervescent and indomitable Suzanne known by all as Suzi; when his hitherto contented life took a different turn.

He had bounded through 50 years of an unfettered existence working in places that didn't feel like any factory or office you might know. A universe largely comprising five star hotels set in manicured gardens, with fine wines, fabulous foie gras, and outrageous flower arrangements, speckled with well heeled customers in which the anticipation of their needs was paramount.

After growing up in Bath he had become an hotelier who delighted in operating some of the very best of Britain's hotels, winning hotel of the year prizes along the way, before founding with some like minded chums his own specialist hotel operating group. Ending up in London he presided over an empire of a dozen or so glamorous hotels which featured architecture of the grade one variety, decadent décor, period fixtures in capability parkland surroundings, and food of the highest standard. His was an untroubled workplace.

Taking time out along the way to invent the truly iconic, deep blue, skittle shaped, Ty-Nant mineral water business and then a niche adult soft drinks company he became an entrepreneur without ever knowing it and a role model for many a novice hotel student along the way.

Then things changed.

Foreword

This is a true story. It offers a unique insight into the difficulties that someone suffering from a major illness has to endure.

Nothing can prepare you for the moment when your closest relation or dearest friend hits a period of ill health which permanently diverts the course of their life. It will affect your life too. By reading this transcript you will have a much better insight into the disadvantaged world that you will both be united in.

Try to read it quickly and be amazed, but as it's no page turner- I recommend you take ten treacle thick pages at a time and pause for breath. Read it slowly and be enlightened.

Michael Philpott

Some Comments from the Critics

"Writing is a much better occupation than hotelkeeping!" - Dominic Walsh, 'The Times'

*** *** ***

"When faced with this sort of experience, suddenly life's little miseries seem so trivial. It will give a lot of people a new look at their lives and I thank him for it" - Stuart Harrison, 'Caterer and Hotelkeeper'

*** *** ***

"Whenever the author has crossed my path, he has always had a positive effect on me. This script is no exception. The positive mindset may be no great surprise, but the reminder to us all as you get well into your 'career tunnel' to look after yourself better, and enjoy the process, not just blast on, head down toward an end result, is one, I'm sure not only I will take from these words" - Malcolm Lindley, Chairman 'Estate Agents Guild'

Robin Sheppard wrote this book without notes, records, secretary or the use of his hands.

To GB and SMRC

All proceeds from the sale of this book will be given to the GBS society to help fight the illness and raise funds for further research.

Contents

"Incredible, indefatigable, intelligent, ingenious, indelible, incandescent" - Peter Jewkes, 'The Fountainhead', Spanish Correspondent.

*** *** ***

"It's a great read, sad and funny. The piquancy of the humour sits right up there with Tony Hancock in the Blood Donor when he asked for a badge to be inscribed, 'nothing pretentious, just they gave that others might live'" - Andrew Mourant, 'The Independent'

*** *** ***

"One of those God sent things that makes you re-examine and reassess your own personal life, motives, aims, ambitions and fears… Overall, a humbling event perhaps, but with the friendship and support of those you love coming to the fore Sheppard counts his blessings... for each and every one of them helped him through his ordeal" - Ali Vowles, 'BBC TV and Radio' Broadcaster

CHAPTER ONE
WINTER OF DISCONTENT

It was one of those breath condensing in front of you cold, sombre days that was there for no other purpose than to prelude Christmas. The local shops were running out of mincemeat and brandy, the scrawniest fir trees were being dragged along pavements by even scrawnier children and conversation was dominated by charity fundraising bucket holders exhorting all passers-by to 'give generously'.

The lack of daylight after three-thirty cast a jet black curtain across the street as I carried my clementine and walnut laden shopping bag up the pathway to the front door and peered at the candles alight in the front window. The tree was up and the cards hung. It should have been a view to make Scrooge weep.

It was the 19th December and I had started to experience a stabbing pain in my back. Pins and needles had begun to affect my senses,

I was losing feeling in my stomach; there was a heaviness in my arms and legs. I had a dry cough. I felt tired and assumed that the flu was coming.

The following day blurred as I noticed a remarkably rapid reduction not only in my powers of alliteration but also in my motor function. An ever escalating sense of agony was growing throughout me, emanating from my spine. Ordinary everyday events like blowing my nose or picking up a telephone became monumental tasks. Every reflex and sensation was draining away. Driving down the motorway in the early evening took great concentration and several stops. Staying in the correct lane was a challenge in itself, so I slowed right down to mask the erratic steering. This was going to be the mother of all colds if the hacking cough and drowsiness were anything to go by.

When I reached my destination, in the spa town of Bath, I was sweating and my walking was uneven and hesitant. I did not feel safe to drive again, so of course ignored my own sage advice and went off to a nearby office the next morning. It didn't last long! The room seemed to be spinning, I kept keeling over like a drunken sailor...why, I even missed the first coffee break.

There was no option but to cancel appointments and get back to bed; somehow the car got me there.

I was staying upstairs in my father's house and tried to ring my GP. After six abortive attempts to get hold of him, I was able to describe my conditions but this was insufficient to merit a home visit. So, placebos all round! He prescribed painkillers. The iceberg had struck the transatlantic liner, and his emergency procedures dictated a brisk shuffle of the deckchairs.

My breathing became irregular, I felt intermittently faint and then quite lucid.

By mid-afternoon, I could no longer walk. Somehow I had gotten out of bed determined to get to the loo. I fell across the dressing table, steadied myself and headed for the door.

I got to the landing, little realising that these were to be my last steps. Rather like Mutley, the Wacky Racer from those classic cartoons, I had run over the edge of the cliff and although my legs were still going round, there was no longer any ground below me.

At that highest point of suspended animation all was still and serene. I remember thinking to myself "Shep.......you're in big trouble".

I crashed to the ground face upwards and there I stayed....... and stayed. Still desperate to pee, help was needed. Stark naked, save for a nearby Nokia 3210 to spare my blushes, I tried to send out an SOS on my mobile phone. The first flurry of texts emanated from my fingertips, which gave up the struggle part way through the exercise, forcing my knuckles to come into their own and take over duties. I was at a loss, not knowing how to describe my malaise without spreading untold panic. I could not speak to anyone because I could not lift the phone upwards toward my mouth. Gravity was in overdrive. Indeed I was only managing to expedite the texts by resting the phone on my hip and tipping my head on one side to see what I was doing.

It was a truly dreadful and terrifying passage of time. A period when the minutes stood still and I despatched a clarion cry for assistance overtaken by the predictive text machinery which turned the simple expression "Help I am in trouble can't move" into a very illuminating "Gely h an go trotter abou note".

Little wonder people ignored me.

I cried out, remembering my father's deafness, at the top of my voice. Dad, bless him, was downstairs watching Countdown and was busy choosing between his vowels and his consonants with the television on full volume. Carol Vorderman stood between me and salvation. Will I ever forgive her for this trespass, or that rubber dress?

I tried to move. Nothing happened. I was completely and utterly immobile.

After what seemed like eternity there was a knock at the front door. Fortunately avuncular Albert our Irish neighbour had come round to drop off some sausages, as you do. Albert heard my cries straight away and, as he climbed the stairs, comforted me immediately with the words "Jesus, look at the state of you. Have you been on the falling down juice?" I apologised for my nakedness while the ever genial Albert decided to take control and call for an ambulance.

Somehow he got me into a pair of bright lemon pyjamas, put a £10 note and mobile phone into my breast pocket and exclaimed "That will see you right."

The ambulance drivers were solicitous in the extreme and put me onto a stretcher, which converted into a chair, and three people lifted me downstairs giving me regular bursts of oxygen. Something was clearly wrong, but what?

It was the 21st of December, I was about to be trussed up like a turkey in the accident and emergency unit of the Royal United Hospital in Bath. How could the shortest day of the year feel so long?

So determined was I to hold onto my breathing, I could not rest, petrified that if I fell asleep I would never wake up. My voice was rapidly getting weaker as the balance between talking and inhaling air grew more tenuous. There was so much I wanted to say, endless questions formulating but which would be left unasked. Each word and every sentence seemed to reduce my lung capacity. This was the real fight, somehow if I could just battle back this paralysing rape as it hammered at my neck, chest, throat and tongue.

To have and to hold....I kept repeating...To have and to hold.

The battle raged for hours, the war ran into days. My captor was gathering strength like a mid-Atlantic hurricane seeking its gateway to carnage.

Burrowing away inside, clearing any sign of resistance until it was ready for the final brutal assault on my constitution. The senior consultant who patrolled the accident and emergency department, like an officious sergeant major, did not tell me what he thought my illness might be. He merely explained that my breathing would probably give out soon and I should not be surprised or alarmed by this. Easier said than done! I was quite attached to my breathing and had no intention of letting go of this much practised skill.

Various appliances had been rigged up around me to help stabilise my condition, the usual suspects were lined up in an identity parade beside my bed including saline drip, blood extraction piping and an applicator to ply me with painkillers. These were the only items that I could identify. The faces of the staff, other patients, and layout of the room were beyond my recall. Those days leading up to Christmas were stolen from me. Time seemed to stand still. Some greater power pressed the pause button and erased nearly three days.

I was inundated with the first wave of nearest and dearest who were struggling to come to terms with what appeared to have happened to me. I wanted to reassure them, to show that I was remaining upbeat despite the confirmation of the seriousness of my condition that my body was supplying me with. There were looks of real concern written across their faces. Whether they wanted to provide this damning endorsement or not, the choice had been removed, no one who came to see me in that time could hide the terror that my countenance induced.

Breathing was getting shallower and more difficult by the hour, then by the minute. I wanted to fight, keep pushing out the old air and gulping down the new. Sliding what air I could in while the alien force was slipping behind my tongue and shunting the oxygen out faster, then faster still.

I could barely talk now. No surrender.... I will.... fight this....The lull started to break. Batten down the hatches. There's a storm a comin' in!

Here comes that moment when you are supposed to see all of your past life before you.

Yes here it comes.....can't breathe, can't speak.....pressure on my lungs, Jesus, Mary....no air, I'm drowning here, help me, sweet Joseph, could you answer this prayer.....gulping, gasping.... distended lips mouthing like a freshly caught trout, eyes rolling in their sockets. I can't breathe, I can't Breeeee....falling, falling, falling. ....all... the way.......down....

It was Christmas Eve, staff were running toward me in slow motion, the lights were going on and off, there was an overwhelming white noise, finally my breathing collapsed, as though I was just dropping off to sleep and that sudden sense of falling took me away. I wanted to shout "Don't fret, it's only a Myoclonic jerk…happens all the time"….but all is rushing, there are trees ripped out of the sodden earth flying past my window, branches flaying….I am leaving…. cheerio…Ta-Ta….goodnight.

I passed out………

Life, real honest to goodness life, with its catastrophes, murders and out of the blue inheritances of inconceivable wealth happens almost inevitably in newspapers. Surely life was not happening to me, not now, not here…so much still to do, so many songs to sing, operas to write and words to say.

I don't want to be dead!

But I just have….died

I think

But if I am thinking, I can't have

So where and what am I now

Open my eyes….listen….smell…there must be clues

Can't,

Want to

Still can't ….all is surreal.

Drifting like tumbleweed down a deserted midwest street...out of control...captured by capricious winds...rolling over then around.... up and beyond any misplaced boulder....falling now...drifting away to different vistas.

Images, cloudy and opaque, flashed in front as if drawn from the deepest fevered vortex.

There were stiff white sheets and pale green walls, dark blue uniforms, powerful extraction fans so high in the ceiling that I could barely see, strip lights in curious housing designed with reflective material as works of art, next to endless panels of off-white rectangles set in the roof. Silver mirror material all warped and bent like fun fair mirrors; twist my head a fraction to the left and there's a bridge, seaside and wooden beach groins, turn a tad to the right and the lights mutate into reflections of motor cars reversing by a hundred kerbs. It was such a kaleidoscopic view ever distorting, created by each millimetric shift of the eyeball, as I looked upwards in search of reassurance.

I kept on staring at the ceiling with an unblinking gaze, unable to see my feet, or the scratches on my hands and arms where tubes had been inserted.

Something is not right about my neck. I don't think it belongs to me.

I can't see or sense my fingertips, or toes. My back has been broken in two, or so it appears.

I can't lift my head off the pillow or move any part of my body, save my mouth which can open and shut like a ventriloquist's dummy, but produces no sound.

So is this heaven or hell?

Which one did the good Lord choose?

Does it really matter, because I feel so abused and abased, so battered and bashed, so comprehensively crushed?

Maybe it is neither, maybe I am still alive, maybe the doctors in this hospital managed to rescue me from the typhoon and just maybe someone has looked so kindly on me that there is a second coming. Why it's a new beginning, a second half, a chance for redemption. There is a possibility that life may start again with alternate rules and a whole fresh agenda.

It is, after all, Christmas Day, I think. How auspicious.

How prescient, what a day to be born again. How finely balanced is that glass by which we judge whether life is half-full or half-empty. Just being alive should provide all the knowledge we need. My glass will always be deemed 'half-full' from now on. Time to start fighting back perhaps, but right now I need assistance and lots of it.

Help was indeed at hand, but the fanfare that ushered it in was not as triumphal as you might expect. Something majestic, even priapic, to mark this reprieve would have been sweet, perhaps a little Beethoven girding our loins with "Ode to Joy" at full volume?

Perhaps not...........

I awoke to the distant strains of Noddy Holder exhorting "So here it is, Merry Christmas, everybody's having fun". Was that mulled wine and mince pies that I could smell circling around this unfamiliar ward?

Where am I, the intensive care unit?

Nurses appeared wearing red antlers and tinsel, blissfully unaware that I had a demon scratching the tip of my nose and was completely unable to do anything about it.

.......And so the next chapter of life began.

Without warning my body had been taken hostage, I hadn't given anyone permission for this to happen, nor was I expecting it, but there was no doubt that I was facing a Second Half.

I was now trapped in my own body.

This was a very different form of imprisonment, where the cell was in the head and the exercise yard was closed. Still there weren't any cockroaches or bars on the windows. In time maybe I could start to plan the escape from Alcatraz, but not today. I had work to do first.

That meant staying alive, for a start.

The autopilot controlling my destiny had been re-programmed with just one target. Descend with alacrity toward the inexorable crash landing, that was the sole instruction.

Any sense of day and night had disappeared, the only way I could tell was by studying the faces looking after me, as some people only worked at night. The evening should have heralded a period when things got quieter, but in the intensive care unit there was no peace for the wicked or the unwell at any time of day or night. The sleep deprivation caught up with me. Noise had become my latest assailant venting torture as any sound twisted and tormented my hearing. The ears had gone into maximum overload as the other senses receded.

There were 27 people in the ward all needing immediate help, each was attached to a number of devices which activated a sound, either when supplies ran out or there was a change in behaviour. It sounded like an orchestra permanently tuning up......Whiz, bang, crash, wallop, plonk, kerpow.......

There was no sign of a conductor to bring them to heel.

Surely intensive care is somewhere you go when you're really, really ill. I don't belong here, I will be as right as rain soon enough. There is some perfectly logical explanation for this minor inconvenience and I will be back on my feet in no time at all........This is such an alien experience. I have been taken captive and morphed into this penitentiary to study absolution.

The layout of the ward was not something I could grasp, images were too vague and transitory to cement in the brain. But I could still count and they moved me seven times from one bed to another as each successive case was admitted to the ward and required a higher priority. Now I knew how those old-fashioned filing systems were supposed to work.

Only I was fulfilling the role of the lonely memo which required attention when it first came in but which mattered less and less when compared with the daily influx of new crises that overtook it.

My body was on its journey determined to get as far away from my brain as it possibly could, leaving a point about halfway up my neck and above relatively intact. Picturing myself like a macabre cartoon of a motorbike accident victim, I imagined that my brain had been placed in a separate pickling jar with pipes leading out from it and feeding into components of my body which lay strewn around the laboratory in abstract kit form; my liver bubbling away in a test tube and my thighs simmering in cider flagons, my arms in Belfast sinks and my back in a basin. There must be a picture guide to this newly fragmented jigsaw puzzle. I don't want to spend the rest of my life with my head in a jar and my body in various buckets.

Interruptions became a new way of life. Change was constant and the only staple part of the staff's diet was adrenaline. So challenging were some of the cases admitted that it took every ounce of their concentration to cope with the pace and intensity.

The new arrivals took precedence, drama upon drama. None were well enough to form any alliance or kinship with. Relations were too concerned with their own nightmares. It was a very singular time. Just when I thought things were starting to slow and stabilise, another one of my faculties closed down. Happiness had gone into hiding, hopefully hidden just around the corner, temporarily out of sight and out of mind. It left a vacuum which was filled with trepidation and bursts of unbounded misery.

In such despair impressions, half formed, were fitted with links that might catch hold of each other. Aided by happenstance, or serendipity, I tried to render some modest coalescence possible, but.....I did not know what to fasten on to in this wasteland....so emasculating, and hostile were my darkest moments.

Like most men I had left the Christmas shopping to the last minute, yes I had wrapped some gifts for loved ones, but while the Sellotape, the scissors, the wrapping paper, the cards and the frankincense and myrrh were all under the same roof they were no use to anyone without assembly.

Worrying about Christmas presents was akin to the irrational fear of being caught in an accident without fresh underpants. Yet in this place of acute vulnerability where life was trying to dodge death by holding onto a gossamer thin thread it was such trivia that dominated.

It was a curious place to be in this state of debilitation. The mind appeared to be intact, the body clearly wasn't.

Messages from my brain to my limbs bounced back like unwanted e-mails, where had my body gone? It still appeared to be there, yet the 'disconnect' was so profound that a new reality had to be accepted and quickly.

I wondered if Surferdudes off the coast of Hawaii felt that kind of 'in body out of body' experience as the perfect wave broke over them and they entered the 'green room' to snake, pirouette and arc toward the shore, atop their beloved surf board. Mine was an altogether drier experience, particularly as I was now under a regime of nil by mouth and the closest I got to water was an ice cube around my lips. It was fearful thirsty in the Sahara of my brain.

Unable to move and without the ability to speak, communication was impossible save the effect on others that my appearance had. I couldn't even control that either. There were several tubes around me, two of which I had watched being pushed into my left nostril. They added a certain elegance to my outfit, the colours complementing my, by now, peppermint pyjamas. The first tube measured a meagre 40 cm but warranted a senior doctor and three auxiliaries to rotate and steer the invader through my nose, down the throat and into the stomach to enable the build up of excess air to be siphoned off.

The second was a more impressive 60cm and took far more twisting by two sets of hands to turn the tip beyond the tummy and into food absorption headquarters. The doctor maintained a dull running commentary throughout with all the inflection of an automated 'I speak your weight machine'. In my mind Murray

Walker was leading the description as into the hairpin bends raced the tube before executing a perfect overtaking manoeuvre through the chicanes, on the way to the duodenum.

A hole had been cut into the lowest point of my neck through which the most important pipe had passed. My lungs rose and fell charged with air supplied through this tube at a very regular pace.

I was plumbed in to a life-support machine, which was intrusive, scratchy, overwhelming and ever so welcome. Without it, if I had been born in another country or a previous generation I would be dead, with it I had a chance.

My thoughts wandered through periods of crystal clarity, into depths of despond, fug and confusion. I came to rely upon the steady rhythm of my controlled breathing for the obvious physical need and as the tempo for my mental mantras, which repeated over and over, "Fight, fight, fight". The beat was steadier than Ringo Starr, and almost as monotonous as one of his drum solos.

My stomach stopped working.

The external manifestation of this illness could be seen by the lack of movement in the limbs and trunk. The internal machinations were more mysterious. The eyelids gummed together reducing or curtailing visibility so that seeing clearly was an event separated by days and only lasting for minutes. My mouth dried to such an extent that I needed fake saliva to be sprayed under my tongue. My bottom went on strike too, which can be useful if you don't have the right change for the station loo in Zagreb on a cold night, but hopeless if it lasts for weeks. Feeling through the hands, other than constant pain had disappeared, awareness of any internal sensation vanished. Hot or cold water on my flesh felt the same as a rough towel. It seemed that a magnetic force had wrapped itself around me and was busy repelling all comers. Yet I craved movement. Any nurse prepared to help me move on my side, rearrange pillows, or adjust the various pipes feeding into my body, became an instant candidate for beatification. I watched them act out their parts in the hospital play through one half open eyelid or the other.

Giving care on a one-to-one basis to critically ill people is quite a vocation.

I'm sure that I would not have the dedication, the steely resolve and the altruism required. But boy did they impress. The staff came from all walks of life, from Spain, the Philippines, Kenya, even Bristol. Some had been born in the road next to the hospital and never been out of the county, much less abroad. All were bound by one shared instinct, to do their very best to keep their charges in the best condition that they could possibly summon. One nurse....one patient.....one agenda.

On an especially harrowing night I overheard the death of a mother who had been stricken by operation after operation. They had failed to stem the internal bleeding and root out the cause.

It was like listening to a ghastly radio play as I could not turn my head to see the characters perform.

The family was dysfunctional in the extreme, and the young daughter had no love for her stepfather. To hear the cries of that poor seven-year-old go on and on as she realised that her mother had died was excruciating. No one, least of all those close to her, could provide comfort or succour.....what a chilling welcome to Cold Comfort Farm.

I thought of friends, and thought of my best buddy who is a doctor. I once asked him how he coped with explaining death to relatives. "It's simple. I just tell them that he or she has died." "Don't you sugar coat it, with a, we did the best we could or they put up a brave fight?" "No, I keep it straight, because sometimes I may have to do three or four in a day. If I give too much empathy to any one case there's less of me for the next hard luck story. I have to protect myself as well as the relatives." This had always struck me as being excessively harsh. Now I understood. His explanation needed context, which was being demonstrated in ample proportions down on the not so funny farm.

I would have felt hungry had my belly not continued to bloat with air, modelling itself on the contours of the nearby Solsbury Hill on which the pop mogul Peter Gabriel once opined in a catchy song.

Why can't everybody understand what I am saying by reading my lips? This is a perfectly reasonable request. I need to turn over. I have become sore in this position and have counted all the panels in the ceiling. My goodness, how well I can stare at things now...., this morphine makes me feel very strange.

Are the doctors getting younger, I thought it was just policemen who did that?

"It may come as a surprise to you but we believe that you have an illness called Guillain-Barre syndrome," said the reassuring doctor, aged 17 3/4. What's that? I wanted to say but the expression in my eye would have to suffice. She was good at reading eyes.

Trying to be concise she listed what she knew about this illness.

It affects about 1000 people a year in the UK.

The immune system gets the wrong message, thinks it is under attack and so attacks itself.

Most patients recover from the illness within two years...but for some it takes up to seven.

It is a slow and exhausting process and you will always be left with a level of residual tiredness.

You should be able to walk again and recover 95% or more of your original faculties.

I'm sure she went on to tell me many more things but I got stuck at the point where she mentioned two years...... this seemed like a very long time indeed.

How can I put this into context? Pain, tears, happiness, joy, laughter and loss were all colours in the past rainbow of experience. Did

I have any reserves in latent suspension waiting to be activated? How do you remove such a vast level of faculty without replacing it with something? Surely there was a way I could cope with this new reality by gaining strength from previous tests. Inject industrial quantities of self belief perhaps? Or maybe now was the time to really understand the family motto "Dum Spiro Spero"? While I Breathe I Hope.

Hope was my mother's middle name and surely everything comes if man will only wait. So waiting for hope to show up would be my new hobby? Now let's be practical here, start with the foundations and build up. Normative needs sit at the bottom of the hierarchy of needs, way below fancy cars and fine holidays, and even further below the state of self-actualisation that one is supposedly searching for to cap the pyramid of our desires.

When you are thrown so wildly off course from the usual aspirations of your selfish life normative needs become the only focus. How you breathe, eat and sleep is so important that you are incapable of thinking of anything, let alone anyone else.

Fear of the unknown causes mankind to be afraid of many things, things like death and public speaking, which absurdly is supposed to rank the higher of the two.

There are many ways to die. Being buried alive is apparently the option most reviled by humans. According to Edgar Allen Poe 'to be buried while alive is, beyond question, the most terrifying of those extremes which has ever fallen to the lot of mere mortals.'

This was to be no apocryphal moment for me. Yes fate had determined to bury me inside my own custom-built coffin. I could not detect six feet of earth on top of my chest, yet the effect on my ability to move from this amorphous state was identical.

Desperate to fight back and break out of this singular cell, the anguish and the gut wrenching melancholy were palpable. But there had to be a way out, best form my own escape committee.

I didn't just need people around me to do good deeds, offer prayers, roll their rosaries or a gospel choir to extol the virtues of born-again religion. I needed Resonance by the bucket load if I was to return from the dead.

The main problem was that the chief supplier of this season's deluxe, must have, everything must go today, special offer Resonance was out of town, leaving me in charge.

Everybody who was close to me wanted to be useful and were, in their own way, as helpful as it was possible to expect them to be. That was all anyone looking in on the internee could do though. Unless I took charge and set my own pace and agenda the building blocks would never be put in the right order. This may sound ungracious or vain; it is neither. It is just what life does when one person's destiny is knocked so far out of line, putting a tangible distance between you and other people. Those closest were still seemingly adjacent, but they weren't in the house with me anymore, they were outside looking in. Concern was etched over their every facial expression. My new role was to be the object of this concern. I had been absented from smelling the roses in the garden, and no amount of protestation would let me outdoors again. You can feel the presence of your nearest and dearest, their scent, their warmth and their passion. It just does not taste the same. Too many of your six senses have been removed or terminated for there to be valid comparison any more.

The sense of helplessness is all-engulfing. Apart from being able to move my head from side to side and open and close my mouth and occasionally my gummed up eyes there was no other movement I could initiate or sound I could make. Why should anyone want to talk to me? I could not open up a discussion, voice approval, stimulate debate or tell a witty tale.

Yet the most restorative medicine the nurses could give came from the one-way conversations that they had with me.

There was a system whereby the nurses would cluster and proceed around the ward in small gangs of two or three. Their aim was to check that all vital supplies were getting through.

They used intravenous drip for the water supply, Immunoglobulin to repair the damaged nerve endings, food through the nose, painkillers by syringe, spit by spray and depression suppression by crushed tablet. They would fluff up my bed, straighten my sheets, mop my brow and talk to me. Several were very skilled in the execution of all these tasks but many failed with the latter.

Dignity was not something I had ever considered becoming compromised.

Sure enough though, it had disappeared to the lost property office in record time. The inability to control bodily functions is hardly a shock to those people who live and work in hospitals.

For people like me who are new to the game it is something you can't stop wanting to apologise for.

I am sorry you have to wash my armpits, fit me with a catheter, replace my soiled trousers and apply eye drops to prevent the lids from gluing together. If I could only talk I would tell you how grateful I am.

It really doesn't matter. You have entered a new universe in which the old rules no longer apply. No one cares about the sensibilities, the vexations, or the inappropriate behaviour because now it is entirely the opposite. Making a mess of the bed clothes is absolutely the done thing, it is appropriate and apposite. Discard at a stroke 50 years of prejudicial learning to establish the difference between right and wrong. Forget what constitutes dignified behaviour, and don't spare the horses.

This metamorphosis is quite a leap of faith, yet so inevitable that you simply should not waste time thinking that there may be an alternative. Whatever my dignity used to be no longer is. It is an ex-dignity, it is deceased. Like many a parrot before it, my dignity has fallen off its perch.

Fear had out-manoeuvred dignity and was now all-pervading, mainly a fear of the unknown but particularly a fear of likelihood and statistics.

A more senior doctor came to see me proffering some research from Japan and Denmark. She explained that she was pleased that I did not appear to have contracted polio, which was a fright in itself, but the statistics in her research garnered from The Lancet made her believe that I was unlikely to walk again.

This information was unwelcome and unfeeling. You could have knocked me down with a feather, if I hadn't been lying flat on my back anyway, when she imparted this news. You could have tried tickling me with it too, but you would not have got very far.........I was suddenly in the most bellicose mood.

You see, there are two types of Guillain-Barre and in true fast food restaurant style I had decided to "go large".

This meant that I had the axonal variety of the syndrome, which damages the nerve endings more thoroughly than its less capricious sister.

The myolin which protects the nerves, a bit like the grey plastic insulation around your domestic copper electrical wiring, is stripped away more vigorously with the axonal strain. This leaves exposed nerves to short circuit each other, adding to the mayhem. Apparently, I was an unusual case because of the pace of the decline. It is more common for people to worsen over a two to three-week period.

It is also much more usual for the syndrome to attack only part of your body, say from the waist down. It very rarely strikes so completely and at such velocity.

What exactly do you say to a doctor who was just told you that you are unlikely to walk again?

Well I took the hostile route and in the faintest whisper hissed back that I most certainly would walk again. I was cross and had lost the diplomacy to be polite.

The anger that coursed through my veins was a good thing, it told me that I had the will to fight, and that I was not going to give in to this illness. I was absolutely determined to make as full a recovery as possible. I kidded myself that my message had been received, the rant remained private. No one could understand a word I was trying to say.

The assured, urbane doctor went on to enlighten me. There was more demising to do. Things were not bad enough yet. Apparently the next 16 days of this attack on your nervous system are the worst once your breathing has collapsed.

There is a period thereafter when the deterioration bottoms out, literally in my case. Then you begin the ascent from the very foothills of Kilimanjaro to the top of the peak as slowly as any novice mountaineer without sherpa, roadmap or woolly socks. The oxygen supply problem is a reversal of that experienced by people climbing rock faces. As you recover your ability to consume and process air improves.

In cricketing parlance I had taken a hit for six. Mentally I was all over the shop. My inner family sanctum had put their lives on hold. I had ruined their Christmas as well as my own.

My indefatigable partner Suzi had abandoned her family festivities and made a beeline for my bedside. And there she stayed offering pragmatic, unfailingly cheerful and very firm support. Without her devotion I would have been an emotional cripple, with it I was just a wreck.

The effect on my family was in a way more difficult to cope with than the effect on myself. Watching my eldest teenage son Sam recoil in horror at his first sight of me lying prostrate, unable to articulate the shock as if he had just witnessed a horrendous train derailment, was hard. George, my first wife, and Charlie my youngest son, bless them, were desperately trying to work out what practical help could be provided to make life more tolerable for me and remove pressure behind the scenes by taking care of my then 89-year-old father.

Dad wasn't strong enough to go out shopping for himself and his own health was in such a parlous state that my malaise was bound to have the wrong effect.

Suzi's two adult children came down from London with their best friend James. Charles and Amanda just burst into tears straight away. Mark you I did look especially ill that day as my complexion had apparently turned to a funereal shade of grey.

I wanted to cry too, but crying inside would have to suffice as my eyes were so gummed up. Grandpa Charles, Uncle Tom and Dickie Blo were wonderfully constant in their affections and companionship; being particularly helpful by taking more than their fair share of visiting duties and assisting behind the scenes.

Another friend of mine who enjoyed the exact same spelling of my name, Robin Sheppard, came to visit.

Armed with photographic libraries, including holiday snapshots, pictures of trips to the Arabian Gulf, wild nights of excess in Paris and most spectacularly the new fence being put up around his son's postage stamp front lawn, he droned on and on. I was usually happier if the creosote was applied to the timber before construction and might have ventured this opinion in a less life threatening environment. Robin had absolutely no understanding of what was needed by a seriously ill person at such a critical point. The expression 'intensive care' had provided not one clue to him and his well-intentioned but misguided behaviour was so out of kilter that I was unable to cope.

This visit was particularly instructive because it taught me that I wanted people to come and visit but was incapable of maintaining concentration for more than ten minutes at a time. Or five minutes if fences were on the agenda. Some might say that I had never been particularly tolerant of people when I wasn't feeling social but the yawning and closing of one eye or the other brought my boorishness to new heights. Pleasantries and good manners had their place for sure. Right now they had been evacuated to their very own safe house, for their protection and a spot of re-programming.

Food in the intensive care department was something I could only picture. All sensory delights were denied, no awareness of seasoning, flavour or texture was available. Meals came out of a sickly green, soup-like mixture from a syringe, and were injected into the tube in my nose to bypass the stomach and head straight into the duodenum. The stomach had only agreed to air removal, not consumption during its sabbatical. Other patients were fed in a similar fashion, no Red Mullet Mousseline with Tomato Coulis in sight, far less a crisp dry Sauvignon to enhance the piquancy.

When you are really ill it is most likely that you will die from pneumonia in the early onset rather than the disease for which you were admitted to hospital in the first place. This entitled an army of Physio Terrorists to appear at your bedside at will, moving with the stealth of the Spanish Inquisition.

Without warning, just as you felt you had come to terms with the discrepancies in your breathing caused by excess mucus, one of these ferocious girls would clamber across your chest, open the flap in your neck, and attach what felt like the middle bit of a bagpipe to the hole where your tracheotomy was.

Then in one deft movement, turn you on your side, shake you vigorously, and squeeze the bagpipe in and out like a demented piper whilst explaining "that's a good bit of gunk gurgling away on your chest, cough for me now, that's it, go on, one more!"

These interruptions punctuated my day five or six times. The rest of the time I was half awake and half asleep, drifting randomly from night to day. Imagining some murky lagoon where the mist sat low over the waves and I kept afloat, bobbing up and down like flotsam, shipping too much water, struggling for air. The analgesics masked my perspective of reality behind a façade of hallucination and detachment.

There may have been a sharply defined world out there but I could not see it, existing in a semiconscious Arcadian dream where all faces were silhouettes, all noises muffled and all colours smudged. Indeterminate voices whispered nonsense as spectres and ghouls made merry with my heart.

It is a desolate wasteland in the mind when the palliatives take hold and erase your concentration, cutting you loose from your moorings to drift through colours and clouds, vapours, eddies and whirlpools. In one rare moment of clarity I pictured a man arriving at the Voluntary Euthanasia Superstore, to keep his appointment with his maker.

After showing him to his room he was asked his favourite colour so they could set the shade over his bed before being posed the question everyone should have their answer ready for...

"What kind of music would you like to die to?"

I know, do you?

Later that day a kindly nurse had told me that she knew how to help me hear my own voice. This at a time when I couldn't talk at all seemed very strange. Rather like one of those keys that you use to peel back sardine tins, she curled back the flap in my neck, tweaked my vocal chords with a blade and invited me to speak. Something came out, a bit like the high pitched toy sound that clowns make when they swallow helium from a balloon. That was the good news.

The bad news was the smell. I smelt death.

The combination of dryness and dust from old parchment blown up my nostrils by the devil himself made me startle. It had seemed such a kind and considerate suggestion by the nurse, yet here I was, truly scared. Not only did I think I had seen the other side, but I had smelt it too. I could hear the Adagio by Albinoni swirling, accompanying the movement of my ashes, and as the violin strings transported me, I felt icy cold. It was acrid, yet sweet, centuries-old but so vivid and current. Death was dancing on my tongue, a jig of delight perhaps, mocking my many human failings. Chilling in the sharpness of the image … and suddenly he was gone.

Little did I know that we were to meet again later in the year but at that very moment I wasn't accepting visitors, far less such hostile ones who had not been invited; you can clear off, I am not ready yet. The euthanasia guys are next door, go and ask them their favourite colour.

Whilst jousting with the devil made time pass more quickly the rest of life was passing by much faster. From keeping the finger on the pulse of my business to absolutely no awareness of the wider world was car crash quick. There was plenty of work to do, many people to contact and projects to get on with even without this interruption. Now there was the much bigger complication of handling inquiries from those to whom my absence was a real nuisance, as well as trying to explain what had happened in a succinct fashion to current friends, long-lost buddies, relations and well-wishers.

Suzi became everything to me. She was my ears, eyes, hands and mouth. She found time to become team cheerleader too and in trying to make sense of all the surrounding nonsense decided it would be a good idea to arrange visits by spreading out the numbers as best she could. Calls were transferred to her mobile phone and she garnered e-mail addresses to send out a regular "Round Robin" update, pun intended.

Rather than allow the flurry of visitors who dropped in to see me over the first few days to continue, strict instructions were issued from our version of air traffic control. Like planes hoping to land at Heathrow visitors would have to taxi lest they clash with each other or the time-consuming processes that the nursing staff put me through.

Unfortunately when sending out the first e-mail Suzi announced that she was now running my 'dairy'.

Requests for two pints of gold top went straight over our heads for the first few days until we realised the dyslexic howler.

This did not augur well for explaining, let alone spelling or pronouncing Guillain-Barre correctly. By the way, it's Ghee-Yan Bah-Ray.

Then I got a visit from the pain police. Yes, the hospital had an entire department dedicated to the study and relief of pain. Their leading Professor, Michael, complete with silver beard and gravy spattered tie, introduced himself as nonchalantly and sweetly as the arrival of apple blossom on a sun-kissed May morning. There was real kindness in this man, a reassuring tone to his measured words, and a Pandora-like ability to open my mind with a vocabulary previously unknown. Admittedly conversations were very one-sided to begin with, more monologue than verbal discourse but his insights and past experience provided succour and balm.

Layer upon layer, he started to build up a vivid picture of what it was like to be cast adrift inside this illness. His visits were regular, and supremely helpful. The body may have been comatose but my mind was desperate for direction.

He crafted words and sentences like a man working a block of wood, plying his rasp along the grain one moment then gouging feverishly the next. Michael had a remarkable ability to break complex emotions and behavioural study into memorable headlines. In such a woolly setting he provided clarity, reassurance and a sense of purpose. Not so much a strategy for recovery, more a hitchhiker's guide to redemption.

These visits were in stark contrast to those of the gaggles of student doctors let loose across the ward. The unusual nature of my complaint meant that I was a box office attraction. There is quite a phenomenon in which a senior physician will assemble a posse of enthusiastic, dishevelled young people in white coats and talk to them openly about the patient in front of them as though that patient does not exist. They called it the 'committee rounds.'

Amongst the most recent things to disappear from my system were my reflexes. As if to punish me for this crime student doctors were encouraged to lift my leg from the thigh upwards, strike me just below the knee with one of their specially adapted hammers as hard as possible and watch in astonishment as absolutely nothing happened.

So they went on to attack my ankle, elbow, wrist, and anywhere else they could think of to witness the same compelling lack of movement.

As non-events go it was a good one, mirrored by my own muteness and inability to offer the merest hint of a bodily reaction. This stirred fresh animated discussion amongst the sartorially challenged committee, who confirmed what a hopeless case I was.

If the hierarchy of life resembled a food chain their judgements, delivered in such a dismissive and insensitive way, would have demoted me to the level of a not so fresh cabbage.

Vegetables have feelings too, you know, and I wanted to cry like an onion! Yet I comforted myself with the knowledge that a committee is, after all, a group of the unwilling, picked from the unfit, to do the unnecessary. This made me feel better, particularly because it was not fair or reasonable.

Fair and reasonable were no longer part of my daily vocabulary. They had been replaced by words like nugatory and cadaverous.

My hair was starting to fall out at an alarming rate, clumps of redundant silver decorating the pillow each morning. My bones were under threat of wasting like my muscles and therefore needed drugs to arrest this decline. Pain continued to escalate as my tolerance dropped through the zero mark into negative territory. So I was given a TENS machine to provide an ameliorating electric impulse up and down my spine. Pregnant women will testify to the efficacy of the TENS system for suspending awareness of pain. It doesn't make it go away but it does at least help screen some of the more malicious nerve tingles like a junk mail filter.

There was some perverse news about my skin. While the skin on my face was becoming blotchy and parched caused by lack of direct sunlight and my inability to process my own waste;It was blistering away as rapidly as if someone had set fire to it. The skin on my body which until recently had been ripe with patches and scabs was clearing up. The psoriasis was leaving its home because it needed a strong immune system to thrive. I was no longer an attractive landlord. My bottom meanwhile, in an act of genetic modification, developed a satellite.

Yes, I grew a second sphincter and felt surges of panic as each time I wanted to pass a stool, number one valve remained trenchantly closed and the new portal transmitted 'mission accomplished' messages back to my disbelieving brain.

While all these problems, minor in themselves, were aggregating I was accumulating friendships with some of the nursing stars of the intensive care department who would remain constant in their companionship for months after leaving their care.

I think it was more than pity.

This 50th year, superficially so cruel in cutting me down to a very small size, was starting to offer me an insight into the halcyon bits of human nature that I always hoped would exist but which I had never gathered the evidence to demonstrate before. It was a veritable curate's egg of a year, indeed.

There were such clear signs that I had hitherto evaluated life with entirely the wrong gauge. This event had triggered such a tectonic split in the living experience that I was now embarking on a new second life on a separate coastline.

The sea of loss would always be there, cold, grey and as unforgiving as the Atlantic from which this storm had come. Yet the old order of things was gone for ever and the game of two halves was starting its next act with a fresh purpose.

Down in the murky depths of this massive intrusion into my wellbeing there was a relative plateau; it lasted about a week. There is a lot to be said for plateaus, they offer familiarity and enable you to become accustomed to your new found circumstances. The fact that those circumstances were so absolute, so petrifying, and so barren was not important. The elevator was in the basement and could not descend any further. It brought new meaning to the thought of 'deep joy'.

During this time the caring team experimented by increasing passages of time in which my breathing became less reliant on artificial support. They were trying to kick start my air consumption to make me independent again. Very short periods to begin with, measured in moments, became a little longer each day. My stomach returned to duty, reluctantly and completed a half shift. It had become swollen and distended, constantly refilling with air. Now the pot bellied pig profile began to defuse like a slow puncture.

The vocal cords were still mute, but I practised exaggerated enunciation, and those who spent the most time with me learnt, by lip reading, how to interpret more than one word in three.

Yet my limbs and muscles carried on with their route march to redundancy, because there was no movement, so while part of my body was considering an about turn the rest remained in the exit marked stage left. Target practice beginning on an archery field resembles the initial process. Concentrate on the bull in the middle of the body. Keep hitting that part of the target and your cumulative score will keep rising; your stomach, spine and trunk.

To achieve full recovery though, the analogy moves to the pub where you need to finish your game with doubles around the outside of the dartboard. This can become a kind of 'never-land' in which your fingertips and toes may remain isolated for years, if you can't reach the 'double out' you will be stuck until your whole being can become united again.

The point of intensive care is to stabilise patients as quickly as possible so that they can be transferred into a specialist ward to make way for the next critical case.

It was like the railway station at Crewe, an impressive structure in itself and somewhere many people would frequently rush through but it was no corner table at Fortnum and Mason from which to gently while away the day.

I fervently believed that as I was unable to do anything for myself I should stay in intensive care, hoping that by divine intervention I would awaken, one fine day, totally cured. The authorities knew better and the boot camp regime began in earnest.

The concept of physios trying to get movement out of a paralysed person may seem absurd, but that did not stop them coming each morning to coax me back into once familiar positions. It was vital work because there is so little that can be done with GBS sufferers by medicine or infusion. Time and exercise are the only certain remedy. I tried to join in as much as I could, but every piece of exercise created untold pain. I was plied with drugs to lessen the anguish but this only served to reduce my squealing down to the level of a fractious banshee.

How disconcerting for the team to have their mitigating handiwork met with volleys of invective and tirades of rejecting noise. Articulate I was not. So messed up were the signals from nerve end to brain that primal screaming was my only tongue.

A new antediluvian language was being fabricated in the recesses of my vocal factory. Normal expressions like Ouch, or Urgh were too ambitious.

Cognitive thought was a rarity so finding appropriate grunts in lieu of language was as likely as striking gold on your first pan handle.

Better to imagine the world's worst audition for the job of backing vocalist to Manfred Mann's greatest hits… a veritable fusion of Doowaps, Doowadiddys, Dididums and Didiyes being sung by an urban fox on heat with the amplifier on distort… or perhaps not. It's too depressing a thought! And thoughts and depression were in the process of becoming totally entwined.

Depression is an almost inevitable consequence of GBS so various concoctions were applied until the optimum combination was deemed appropriate by the doctors. This took the edge off many things, particularly excessive fear, but eliminated the emotions that exist at either end of the spectrum.

It was a bit like removing both black and white to leave a palette comprising marginal changes in shades of grey. This certainly stops you getting too depressed, which is the upside.

The downside is that optimism is lessened, joy and euphoria are removed and you trundle along in the middle lane of the carriageway.

Rational fear should dominate. Fear of letting people down, of never realising the potential that life seemed to have guaranteed when boyhood was so rich of promise and expectation, or of missing your own funeral, of being permanently disabled or, even worse, of voting for the Liberal Democrats in a grave error of judgement.

Yet rational never answered the call.

Opposite anxieties took centre stage, trifling details about minutiae cramped the brain. All set against the certainty of my placement, flat on my back, six feet underground, denied energy, awareness and hitherto familiar reactions.

The auto immune response system was in complete anarchic control, dividing and conquering my constitution in its rampant arrogance on a blind destructive path.

The narcotics ensured my thoughts were surrounded and insulated by 'Velleity', like an orbit in which a series of mild desires, wishes or urges were deemed too slight to lead to action.

When the first 16 days, post breathing collapse, had passed and the proverbial oil tanker had slowed before starting to turn around there came a warning.

We won't be able to keep the bed available for you for much more than a month when you will transfer into the neurology ward, I was informed. The experience will be like falling off the cliff at Beachy Head. The contrast between intensive care nursing where there is one nurse per patient to a department where there is one nurse for two bays of patients would hit me hard.

You probably won't like it to begin with!

"Wonderful/heart rending/funny/deeply sad/thought provoking/emotionally powerful.......and yet so pragmatic" - David Gledhill, Regional Editor 'Bristol Evening Post'

*** *** ***

"A tale of physical incapacity told with such mental energy that it is completely absorbing. Two things strike about the author's ability to deal with 'that year' and all of its horrors and frustrations. First, that he was able to give and get so much from all those who came into contact with him and second his sharp eye for the ridiculous – usually turned inwards. What happened to Sheppard has already had a huge impact on me; his telling of his own perceptions is a revelation" - Willow Corbett-Winder, 'Tatler'

*** *** ***

"This is a highly amusing and illuminating recovery story, accompanied by moments of sombreness and despair. Such powers of memory, deliciously told" - Marie-Claude Sable, 'Etampes', Paris Correspondent

CHAPTER TWO
OUT OF THE FRYING PAN

Sure enough, after 30 days I was transferred out of intensive care because I was no longer sufficiently ill. And was placed into a neurological rehabilitation ward where they seemed completely unfazed by my lack of animation.

Patients with the movement of an Egyptian mummy waiting to be embalmed were evidently a way of life, to the nurses and care workers who were to become my guardians and best friends for the next six months. Being paralysed, on a scale of 1 to 10, seemed close to double digits to me. To them it was more of a two or a three. I could breathe for tiny moments of the day unsupported now and that was enough to justify the eviction.

In their infinite wisdom the nurses decided to move me at 2 in the morning on a Saturday night. I felt as though all the emotional crutches had been taken away at the same time, plus we had not stopped off for a greasy doner-kebab on the way, which is what men normally do at 2 in the morning after a saturday night. The new ward was full of old people. At least that was how it smelt. I had no expectation of what a neurological ward would encompass. Principally it was where people who had strokes went, after the first stroke had struck them down, to recover. Or, and nobody ever talked about this, to wait for the second stroke which if it came too soon after the first could be really damaging, often fatal. I didn't sleep that night, or the next.

It took days to come to terms with my new surroundings.

They gave me a bed in the corner of the ward where I should have been able to keep an eye on all the other patients. Keeping an intermittent eye on them was all I could do, I couldn't sit up, let alone stand, and my power of speech was still akin to the scoring of sandpaper on glass.

The job description said that I was to be the new toll bridge "teller", collecting fees from all those who accessed or egressed the ward because my lumpy bed looked over the other five bays.

I could also see down two adjacent corridors and through an internal window over the L-shaped reception desk. This bed offered the most panoramic view of all 'goings on'. It left very few hiding places for staff, patients or visitors to seek refuge in. In this land of the blind the one-eyed man was king. King of my very own Belvedere!

Strange how illness flattens us all and forges the most unlikely alliances.

What's this, a youngster or at least an arrival that doesn't look like grandpa from a Werther's Original advert?

The newly arrived bloke next to me used to stack the shelves at Sainsbury's during the night shift. He was 43 with two children, eight and 5, and a particularly aggressive form of MS. A more giving person you could not hope to meet. Rapidly I became Butch Cassidy to his Sundance Kid. This was our tangent, where two seemingly unrelated people become one through adversity. How we laughed at each others misfortune, finding solace in our ineptitude.

People kept coming and going from the bed opposite us. Had they known its track record none of the patients in that bed would have allowed themselves to be placed there. I watched 12 people die on that mattress right in front of me.

They arrived off some magic conveyor belt which kept churning out an inexhaustible supply of really ill patients with collapsed lungs, strokes down the left, strokes down the right, organ failures, victims of badly administered drugs, negligent diagnoses, bad luck, old age or pneumonia.

The first death was the worst. Nice enough fella.....smoker, stroke, middle-aged and single. Seemed to be stabilising, then it all kicked off about 1 in the morning. Panic buttons, auxiliaries in scramble mode, zombie medics on their 14th hour of the day, curtains flying 'open to shut', wheeling in heart revival machinery... 'Stay with us now, don't let go, hang on in there'... but it was to no avail.

I shall never forget the eerie sound of my first body bag being zipped up in the depth of the night, inch by uneven inch, while the night nurse sucked on her Murray mint... and yes she took her time, you should never hurry a Murray!

It was not a sound that made you feel clean.

In order to have a wash and change clothes it was necessary to be turned. Sometimes this could be done by two or three members of staff working in a trained pattern. If you remember Cleopatra being delivered to the emperor by rolling out of the carpet across the marble floor you will have a good picture in mind.

Now try to imagine Cleopatra being wrapped into the carpet in the first place and you will begin to understand what nursing teams have to do when caring for hopeless cases like me.

They tugged at my arms to create the momentum to flip me onto one side while lifting the bottom sheet across to the middle of the bed, before rolling me back onto my other side and removing the bottom sheet altogether.

Bed baths tended to involve two nurses to wash you with tissues and towels, mild creams and occasionally stringent sprays. They worked around the ward drawing curtains before entering the newly created arena to descend on the next patient. When wiping your bottom they were supposed to spray a certain cleanser over you with the warning "cold spray!" Timing though was never perfect and the spray tended to hit your nether regions long before the warning arrived. It is not the best time for intimate reflection when one nurse has just rolled you onto your tummy while the other tidies up your behind. I suppose we see a mild form of bottom interrogation when dogs greet each other in the street, sniffing each other's behinds with tails wagging in great excitement.

We take this for granted while pretending to ignore the absurdity and obscenity of the pastiche, but this does not prepare you for the level of matter-of-fact attention that your private parts receive, in the course of a nurse's daily work.

Nor does it prepare you for the speed with which you are returned so quickly to normal social etiquette. I wondered what the old Sloane Ranger's handbook would suggest as the most mannered way to show gratitude for having your arse wiped. I must ask the author next time I bump into him, oh no, wait, there it is under Knightsbridge Girls….How to show gratitude… H for help with ablutions just after G for gang bangs…what's that?

G is more interesting than H….oh alright then….after all, aren't we told that Knightsbridge girls are supposed to loathe gang bangs because they 'hate having to write all those thank you letters'?

Getting up and down to the toilet would, in a normal world, be an automatic process in a typical day. For the severely ill it is often simply impossible.

Under the influence of a mild anaesthetic my plumbing had been readjusted.

A bag had been loosely strapped around my right leg just below the knee. A pipe had been inserted into the eye of my penis to carry excess fluid into the bag. This was then emptied periodically through the day. Some young children had come to visit an immediate neighbour in the ward who had experienced the same treatment. With a splendid combination of both spoonerism and malaprop they invented a new term for this device.

Since then I have always referred to it as the Catheteria. A one-stop shop, go for a pee and order a cappuccino at the same time.

I decided it was best to get on amicably with this new appliance and bedfellow. Others around me found this impossible and in their feverish excitement and delusion would wrench the device from their loins in an act of stupefying masochism. Either determined to ignore contrary advice or unable to understand it, grown men would scramble away at themselves like kamikaze lemmings on a one way mission to remove the pipe from their person.

Once inserted, a balloon attachment is inflated inside the body to prevent the tube from being pulled out. Oblivious to the pain which they are about to cause themselves, the yanking accelerates until the howls of excruciation announce the conclusion and the nursing team is summoned to ease the pain and berate the patient for... 'being a pillock'. The balloon is at least ten times the size of the exit route it has just been pulled out of!

I resisted the temptation to follow suit partly because I had no desire to do it, partly because it seemed absurdly painful and of course partly because I couldn't.

Like most obstacles in life you overcome them and you get used to them. Abdicating responsibility for another bodily function just meant the list was getting longer. In time wearing a Catheteria would matter to me and I would want the faculty back but at the present moment it wasn't even inconvenient.

Suzi provided so much succour and practical help with basic ablutions that I do not know how anyone without support from a loved one could manage.

By being at my side so unstintingly she replaced the nurses on countless occasions; or reminded them of tasks forgotten, or worked with them as so often more than one nurse was needed and only one was available. They accepted her as part of the team and came to see her as part of their family and, dare I say it, came to take her help for granted while becoming very fond of her in the process. It was an act of unselfish dedication repeated daily and I remain humbled by her humanity, munificence and pluck.

The physio gathered pace incredibly slowly. I needed to become used to life above the horizontal. The hare's approach was impossible, as I couldn't even keep up with the progress of the tortoise. If you've ever tried moving a dead person you will know how heavy a task it is to move a human being who can't co-operate. Getting anywhere near a sitting up position made me dizzy, three pillows and I couldn't cope with the altitude.

Sitting up on the edge of bed was as intimidating as climbing the Eiger. I had no muscle control, or strength, let alone the ability to stay unsupported in an upright position. So I volunteered for more. You see the NHS only offer physio from Monday to Friday and I did not like the idea of wasting the weekend without making some effort to stimulate movement. The physios were on the whole very agreeable to extra work in return for some pocket money.

After a fight with my insurance company they agreed to fund the cost and I started a grinding daily programme of minute improvement.

What I hadn't appreciated before was that there are in fact two health services, no, not private and public. There is a weekday service and a weekend regime. On Mondays the wards overflow with doctors like a bountiful crop of strawberries spilling out of a punnet.

As the week wears on, the numbers dwindle and by Friday the exodus of expertise completes just before teatime.

Fridays are not a good day to be admitted to hospital as you are unlikely to receive any senior inspection until Monday. Saturdays and Sundays feel like being aboard the Marie Celeste. The worse your command of English the more likely you are to be on duty at weekends.

Ill health doesn't recognise these barriers but they are there, all right, entrenched like some unwritten apartheid. To move away from my amorphous state I needed to keep the body working seven days a week. At best I could manage a half hour session because I had so little strength to call upon, but by building up each day I was eventually able to manage more than one daily burst of activity. Day after day, after day we would go through the motions as I tried to demonstrate enthusiasm and desire.

I had to learn the art of getting into and then retaining a sitting position from scratch. My very first attempt lasted three seconds precisely. One week of coercion later I was ready for the next attempt; this lasted 30 whole seconds and provided the most fantastic endorphin-fuelled rush.

Three days later I was ready for the next bash and succeeded in maintaining a position on the edge of the bed for two minutes unsupported.

It was like winning the World Cup and drinking a bottle of vintage Krug all at the same time. From such a lowly position the team dragged me, always raising expectation and finding something positive to say even when all the evidence was negative.

I resembled an egg which needed its own carton in order to remain upright in uniform fashion. Without it I found the line of least resistance and would flop or subside wherever gravity decided to take me.

I was advised to talk to my limbs in order to send messages back from the head to my extremities, nurturing the reflexes back to life.

Well I certainly sent out the messages all right in the vain hope that some amateur radio ham would hear my mayday message, tune in and broadcast a reaction back to me.

This must be how a comedian feels when doing his first gig of stand-up comedy as the warm up for the main act. No one is listening, no one really cares, they just want the guy topping the bill to get on stage and make them laugh. It doesn't matter how good your script is, how much time you spend polishing and editing to fashion a razor sharp performance.

If nobody wants to hear, then nobody will.

One of the things the doctor had told me about, which I hadn't really heard after the two year bit, was about the pain threshold, and how much worse things would get.

I had been reduced from having one to having less than none, everything hurt.

Personally I prefer to have a thing suggested to me, not told in full. When every detail is given the mind rests satisfied and the imagination loses the desire to use its own wings. This is not good with pain. The excruciation of the agony left no room for self perfidy or for the mind to fly. It just kept on sharpening the poignancy, heightening the bitter-sweetness and drilling right through my sense of enforced masochism.

Perhaps I was becoming engulfed in 'Thanatophobia', which is a morbid dread of death apparently universal in all except those living on Mount Olympus. I couldn't see Olympia or any Greek Gods but I could see daffodils as they started to appear outside the grubby windows of the ward. This made me happier.

Some days the birdsong would cut across the acoustic medley of buzzers and bleepers and alarms that formed the daily cacophony. Some days we even saw sunshine too, but no hint of a God.

Pathos was everywhere, sad stories in front of your eyes of patients who did not know where they were, and worse still relatives who did not care. As spring came upon us and the first tiny shoots of recovery in my body started to take hold I felt like the elder statesman of the ward. If only because I had been there longer than anybody else and knew how slippery the ropes could be for the new recruits.

Each day I witnessed a vocabularical waltz between old Charles who was on his 4th stroke and his estranged wife who like clockwork appeared at five to 10 each morning armed with her local newspapers. She was welcomed by the most vicious barrage accusing her of being late, forgetting his newspapers, being wanton, slovenly, and disloyal. She deflated this attack with her calmness and serenity, reminding Charles that she was five minutes early, she had his newspapers and she still loved him very much in spite of him being the most cantankerous old bugger she had ever met.

To say that Charles was confused would do him a disservice, it was worse than that. His hearing was very poor, memory poorer still and his will to die was failing.

He would set off from his bed destined for the toilet but by the time he got to the doorway of the ward he could not remember why he had set off in the first place.

One day the social worker came to assess him. She pulled the soundproof curtains around his bed and began asking him some questions. Charles could only conduct conversations at full volume so everybody else had no choice but to listen in.

'Do you know what year it is?' she inquired.

'2003,' he bellowed. 'Higher, higher,' said the assembled audience of patients and nurses, trying not to listen in.

'Well, I am not so sure, maybe it's 2004,' Charles boomed. 'Higher, higher,' said the now enthralled game show devotees, giggling as they could no longer choose not to hear.

'Well, I think we've just had Christmas so maybe it's 2005,' said Charles to the most enormous cheer, wolf whistles, clapping, foot stamping and general revelry.

I had been able to witness this vignette while propped up. After what felt like months I was beginning to sit up supported by two pillows, but the physio team wanted more. Their target was to get me into a wheelchair; some days I doubted whether this would be achievable but it didn't stop me trying. To get there I had to pass my hoist proficiency test so that I could be lifted, like cargo from a ship's hold, high up into the air and rotated over the edge of the bed to be deposited onto trolleys, chairs or trestles before being winched back later.

The hoist came in a bilious green colour and was tucked under my back and up through my legs. An electric pulley was winched down from a track in the ceiling and clipped onto the hoist.

Often this was the highlight of my day, particularly as it allowed me to view the ward from a completely different angle. The joy of sitting upright fully supported even if temporary was a very real reminder of the liberty which I had so completely surrendered.

Unfortunately it also offered a view of big John who occupied the bed directly across the ward.

John had suffered his second stroke and somehow had managed to climb over the metal barriers which sat on either side of his bed only to hit the floor with an almighty thwack, breaking his arm and dislocating his collarbone in one fell swoop. He was not an attractive man and had become prone to cussing and spitting. If his own plight had not already made him miserable, then the arrival of his family was sure to do it for him. In one of my least charitable moments I christened them the world's ugliest family or the WUF's for short. A more unsavoury, malodorous and incipiently nasty group of people you could not hope to meet.

This was a bit rich coming from me; chiding them for being unattractive when I was a 'Charles Atlas Before' advert with alligator skin, bald patches, feet shaped like inverted spoons and fingers that resembled the claw in the catch a cuddly toy arcade machine at the end of Yarmouth pier.

An eldest son, four daughters and one wife who had all evidently finished with the Atkins diet, were now feverishly consuming "The Sumo Wrestler's Guide to Weight Gain". They never engaged in eye contact or conversation with any of the other relatives or patients in the ward.

They constantly harangued and bickered with the hospital staff; were ungracious in the extreme and managed to get John's status relegated from one of sympathy to simmering contempt, crying wolf far too often, on his behalf.

Resentful of the condescending way in which they were being treated, the staff queued up to avoid looking after him. The soap opera continued for several weeks but I grew tired of this little cameo and determined to intervene. Without uttering a word between us John and I developed a sign language using nods and winks, even the occasional smile so that I knew when he was genuinely in trouble and really needed help.

Some unwritten script entitled me to act as arbiter on his behalf and bizarrely he would receive attention if I indicated to the nurses with nudges and grimaces that this time his request was genuine. Eventually he was transferred to another hospital, more akin to hospice, and was promptly replaced by a man whose troubles put everything else into perspective.

Tom had Motor Neurone disease.

When first told that I had been diagnosed with GBS I was delighted because I hadn't been told that I had the same illness as Tom.

You see my aunt had died from this slow, simmering, truculent illness, and in my naïveté I thought somehow it might have been genetically transferable. In the circumstances my lack of knowledge was inexcusable really. Yet there I was welcoming GBS like some lost friend solely on the basis that it wasn't what I had most feared.

Of course it wasn't long before I fully understood what GBS was all about.

Tom deserved better than that from me, he deserved better from life too. No one should have to suffer inside such an elongated death. He was a brave and noble man, stoical, fastidious and apparently completely lacking in self-pity. I saluted him then and applaud him now.

On the Move

Often the best moments came through surprise. One was on its way to meet me. I had no idea it was coming and didn't think I was anywhere near being ready.

All that polished chrome, rich burgundy coloured leather, go faster wheels!

Yes it's time for the high back wheelchair...

All things are relative of course, so to someone unable to stir their carcass a wheelchair is a tremendous statement of new-found mobility. To immediate family and helpers it offers something to do which allows them to demonstrate their support in a tangible way. It was not easy to remain in. Yet the very fact that my body was being put into and taken out of a wheelchair was therapeutic in itself. I can't say that I looked forward to getting into it because my spine was still too weak to support my body on its own and my arms were unable to provide the ballast to stabilise me once in the chair. My head had to be tethered, my arms strapped over pillows at very specific angles, and my feet secured. It took four people to get me in place, after getting me out of the hoist.

Somehow, each day, those four musketeers levered me into this unsuspecting wheelchair and strapped me down to prevent me collapsing. It was torture, yet just a prelude to even more vertical challenges.

I couldn't walk, and my arms were like two wasted twigs. The adiposity of my body fat was down to Jane Fonda levels and I found the daily grind of trying to recover movement so tiring that I would yawn during exercise. I had lost 3+1/2 stone. The muscle wastage, when idle, diminishes at about 3% per day. I had been lying on my back far too long .My feet had dropped like a ballerina's. Now you may like a bit of Swan Lake, but for me the next objective was learning to stand. Early lessons were to be conducted on a tilt table. I must have seen something like this as a child on black and white television.

Where an enigmatic man, dressed up like William Tell, took aim with a crossbow at the glamorous assistant with an apple on her head.

In turn, she was strapped to an upright tilt table with a similar look of foreboding on her face, but me without the fishnet tights, petrified of tilting more than 45 degrees.

After months of trying we got the table up to the 90 degree mark. It felt as though I was facing downwards, so strange was the sensation of being upright. My arms hurt in this position so I had to have a tray in front of me to keep my hands facing upwards. Every action seemed to have a consequence which involved pain. It never left, always there, gnawing at my resolve.

I had been fitted with hot neuro wiring for the motor enthusiast guaranteed to take pain from 0 to 60 mph, faster than Richard Hammond impersonating a jet propelled plough on Top Gear.

The conclusion was obvious. There was no substitute for simple hard work, if I was ever to get better.

Meantime back in the ward, with a deft rotation of the beds, naughty Norman appeared in the bay next to me. He was about 5' 3, blessed with long flowing white locks loosely arranged in the style of the first Doctor Who.

If ever pyjamas were designed for one single human being it was Norman. A man born to wear Jim Jam's, he had a cute pair of well worn slippers and some well worn stories too. Poor Norman was losing his marbles, he needed help and far more understanding than was available in this ward.

At night a film crew would appear in his mind and hour after hour of in-depth interview would take place, as he asked his alter ego questions. Innocent in the extreme, this was mildly amusing to begin with, but listening to the sadness of someone using an imaginary mobile phone with one voice to interrogate a different illusionary person with a changed accent and pitch became more and more harrowing. He had no recollection of what he had said over the last few moments or hours, nor any awareness of what constituted night-time.

There was some recollection of his youth but a ceiling had come down about 30 years ago to wipe clean the memories in between.

This was his second year of decline through Alzheimer's and living proof of how it is possible to be so utterly alone even when surrounded by people.

From my 'world on a mattress' the days passed, the weeks merged and the snows came and went. Visitors arrived, by the yard. Some recoiled in horror, others brought warmth and joy with them, but still they kept coming. I felt like King Canute, unable to overcome the invasion into my misery; but I realised that talking, or at least, mouthing words forced me to engage with the world, think of wider horizons and laugh at myself. So the visitors became essential to my recovery.

It was on an unsuspecting weekend that David and Milena arrived with a humour so black that my face ached with laughter.

Pushing me out into the atrium coffee shop of the hospital, my arms tied to the sides of the wheelchair, wrapped in swaddling blankets with my head leaning ominously to one side, I looked like and was something straight out of Jack Nicholson's finest cameos. A pamphlet entitled "sex after a stroke" was placed under my chin, below this across my chest a kidney bowl was rested with the phrase, "please give generously" written across its side. Off they tiptoed, leaving me alone as passing relatives tried not to place their small change in my lap, while suppressing their grins.

I didn't mind being laughed at but I did mind being surrounded by catering outlets.

This exposure to food temptation was too much. I had not been able to have a regular meal since admission.

My mouth was positively grateful to have no seasoning or flavour sensation. I had become so unused to such an everyday occurrence that I would need to relearn the skills and pleasure of consumption.

That night David tried to book a table for dinner in over 27 restaurants, all of which were full, before finally finding one with a table to spare. As he confirmed the timing the waiter was surprised to learn that he wanted a table for three, for this was Valentines night (which David had completely overlooked), and as he put down the handset the waiter was heard to breathe softly one condemning word, "pervert". Which of course made his dinner all the more delicious for me.

My previous world of lunch and supper was soon to mutate into a new Northern land where dinner would be at midday, tea at five and Maltesers with Butch and Sundance would take place anytime. Chocolates and sweets were to become our currency, preferably in a stolen moment when no one else was looking or counting our blood sugar level.

Amidst all these nasty manifestations of illness such as strokes and heart arrests there was a quiet and ruthless predator at work. Diabetes is an odious, pernicious invader of our systems borne out of our 21st-century lifestyles. Ignorance is its ally, constantly aiding and abetting. Top tip, don't fill your blood with sugar.

I chose to ignore all this incredibly sensible advice as I lay quiescent on my bed mouthing the words "yes please" to my friend Sundance when asked if I'd like another Malteser. In terms of range I could move my mouth about two inches to either side and one inch up and down. This did not help my chances of catching anything. For Sundance whose legs were wobbly, with arms that didn't work too well, keeping the Malteser bag in an upright position took a lot of concentration. It was quite likely that he would fall over in the process.

Sundance was determined though to get one of these brown sweets into my mouth. It was necessary for him to drop them from a great height to maintain his balance. This did not help target practice or the laundry bill.

At the 12th attempt we managed to get the much loved sweetie into my mouth, but at what a cost. Chocolate blobs were everywhere, in the sheets, on the floor, inside my pyjamas and even two in the bedpan.

Trying to eat cake was almost as difficult as trying to hide the evidence, no matter how strong my denials the residue of crumbs in the armpits would always give me away.

Out of sight is out of mind, though, and as I couldn't adjust my head to look down the bed I could carry on defying diabetes to my heart's content.

One of the consequences of remaining supine is that getting your hair cut becomes hazardous. The hospital employed a roving hairdresser whose job it was to weave between the wards, offering a trim and a rinse to as many customers as she could fit into one day. My hair hadn't been washed for two months or cut for three; the words "bouquet like an Aborigine's armpit" would do little justice to the steamy halo that welcomed this intrepid crimper.

Unable to get me into a sitting position she cut my hair horizontally. The result was memorable for those people unfortunate enough to have to look at me, Boris Karloff would have been proud. As I couldn't look into a mirror I wasn't too bothered initially.

To those people I didn't want to talk to, it became a positive advantage as patients and visitors alike veered off in opposite directions trying to mask their contempt.

This merriment of the mullet continued until an old Sicilian was admitted to one of the beds in my ward. Joe senior had moved to this country more than a generation ago and just experienced a second stroke which had left him unable to speak and more flatulant than any man I had ever met. Admittedly I used to play rugby in the second row with a bloke who was pretty useful in the lineout and even more useful in the clubhouse after the match when asked to produce his party piece.

He could fart at will!

Not just single little slippery fellows either, he could cluster them, broadcast them in stereo and after a few pints of Bass stop all conversation by firing of a salvo from the heart of his bottom which was guaranteed to clear the club bar as well.

Nobody ever asked why he was called Gatling.

Joe's family used to come and visit him in the classic Italian way. First there would be the mommas and the poppas, then the sons and daughters, closely followed by the grandchildren and their babies. No one else commanded such an audience by saying so little, to such a wide variety of relations.

The rest of the patients prayed for them all to stay for as long as possible as their endless chatter in Sicilian/English sounded so peaceful by comparison with the crescendo that we all knew would surely follow when the family finally left en masse.

Just as the last ciao subsided, Joe started to crank up the volume from underneath the sheets. This was Premier league farting, no nationwide conference part-time bottom burping here. Wilfred Owen would have been proud of the onomatopoeia, as the "Rat a ta tat", rolled into the next "Rat a ta tat". I swear I heard a descant in there somewhere. On one particular occasion the man in the bed next to me started singing a record initially launched by the New Seekers but made more famous as the accompaniment to the real thing Coca-Cola advert 'I'd like to teach my bum to sing, in perfect harmony'... Although I confess, it is just possible that these may not have been the exact lyrics, and it might have been me.

Joe's son, Joe Junior, unaware of the opera that took place each night after he had gone home, was overheard opining on the state of my haircut, from across the ward.

After 25 years in this country he spoke a curious mix of English which most closely resembled Stavros the Turkish kebab shop owner made famous by Harry Enfield, thus 'hello everybody' would translate as 'ello peeps'. There was West Country dialect, plenty of Italian and even a bit of North London cockney as Joe uttered the memorable lines... 'Jesus Christ, look at the state of that bloke's Barnet, it's in a right two and eight and no mistake.'

He came over to talk to me.

'Listen mate, no offence but your 'ead is making me sad. I am a 'airdresser, and I fix it for you.' The following day he arrived with his mother and proceeded to give me a tip top haircut. After we had exhausted the usual banter about 'where you go on your 'olidays' Joe started to wax lyrical about his four daughters. It was as though he was announcing the winner of the Miss World competition as he explained to me how wonderful each one of them was in reverse order.

Nothing too surprising about the choice of language to summarise the majesty of each of his girls, as he snipped away he was clearly building up to the crescendo. At last we got to the beauty of the eldest daughter, who like the other three worked with him in the salon. I was expecting a word like Bellisimo as Joe explained, her long dark hair, curvaceous hips, winning smile and that knowing look… 'but my first daughter she is, how you say?... a right belter.'

He wasn't wrong. She was stunning and that was absolutely the last time I ever expect to hear a father describe his daughter so cutely or curiously. His mother ignored us and carried on sweeping up the result of the haircut from the floor.

Life was not just focused on the hair on my head though, there were other hairy bits to consider.

'How is your erectile function?' enquired the immaculately groomed doctor, who had recently given birth to her immaculately groomed baby daughter. An attractive lady with a confidence, quick brain, trim figure and an air of immense capability, she was not the sort of woman you could imagine cracking nudge, nudge jokes with.

This didn't stop me trying a self mocking riposte which fortunately got strangled somewhere in my vocal chords before coming out of my mouth. It was not a question I had considered or encountered before.

I daresay it's a question you may need a few moments to prepare an answer for yourself.

After a fine bottle of claret you might pluck up courage to regale an all-male audience with the rhetorical question that men fear the most from a woman: 'Is it in yet?'

Which is either the ultimate insult, or very funny, depending on your point of view. But that's the ultimate bloke's bit of blokery which binds men together. Put us in a room full of intelligent women and we are not nearly so cocksure.

Do you consider this to be a closed question, implying a single word response? As in 'fine, thank you' or 'disastrous'. Even more damning, I suppose, could be the answer at the end of the multiple choice questionnaire 'don't know'.

Best to go for the more expansive explanation, assume that it is in fact an open question and the doctor has a spare half hour available; and would be delighted if you would pontificate ad nauseam on the vacillations of your Willy.

I decided to go for the medium response and mumbled 'I think there's still a bit of life there'. Which may well have been true, the trouble was at that particular moment I couldn't remember and my body had stopped sending me updates.

Try it at dinner parties, not at the start of the evening, I grant you, but after the pudding course when the cognac is being proffered. It's a killer question and I promise none of the guests will ever forget the evening, or to consult that Sloane Ranger Handbook to check how best to construct their thank you letters. Have a look, it's probably in there under E.

"Do you have to be near death to discover how well you can write? As dear, much loved and now sadly deceased Frank Muir said, the critical thing that writers have to have is something worthwhile to say and a unique "tone of voice". The author lays bare his fascinating and humbling experience. He is undoubtedly a really strong bugger, whose survival instincts run on high octane... with a resonant tone of voice as deep as Paul Robeson" - David Pinchard, President of the 'Frank Muir Writers Foundation'

*** *** ***

"It made me laugh and it made me cry - in fact I am still crying now. I had heard through the grapevine that a big story was coming, a story that dealt with 'being unwell' but never thought for one moment that anyone could write so poignantly if they were THAT ill" - Jane Tapley, 'Theatre Royal' Correspondent

CHAPTER THREE
SPRING HOPES ETERNAL

After the daffodils came Easter, the changing view out of the ward windows, on the few days when warm clear sunshine burst through, was now of scaffolding against tired redundant buildings. Normally clad by sublimely coloured stone in shades of cinnamon the empty rooms and houses were reduced to tawdry ochres, anthracite greys and concrete dust covered piles of rubble. The trust in charge of the hospital's finances, were busy spending money on bigger corridors for all, while awaiting the arrival of their fourth chief executive in three years.

The rose garden beckoned.

This was an area of peace and calm, sheltered from the wind and a sanctuary in which to revive the soul. How I looked forward to those moments, when I could feel the sun on my face, and the spirits rise. The sunshine brought relief and expectancy. The realisation that I might indeed be able to get better surfaced and the determination to conquer the illness became stronger when outdoors.

The garden was in a courtyard, two sides created by the walls of the original 1930s hospital, and the other two by glazed corridors leading to the children's ward opened by the Princess Royal. It was difficult for the wind to circulate too close to the ground and certainly at wheelchair height. No matter how seductive the days of sunshine appeared it was the time of year when bitter cold could cut through the bone, turning what should have been a pleasant afternoon sojourn into ice station zebra. There was a central fountain which provided an ideal birdbath for ravens and seagulls. Around this were four oblongs of exposed earth in which roses of all primary colours had been planted. In true municipal planting fashion the colours clashed horribly.

Who invented the rule that any exposure to civic planting should attack one's eyesight so spitefully?

Garden maintenance was not at the top of the hospital's budgetary concerns so much of the year it lay untended save for the magpies repeatedly raiding the waste paper bins leaving a trail of debris in their wake.

Miraculously the borders surrounding the garden contained herbaceous arrays in which some emotionally intelligent pioneer, blessed with an awareness of how to blend colours and tones, had laid out the shrubs and flowers delicately and with care.

There was the usual mixed bag of benches donated by grateful relatives, dedicated to their departed loved ones. Above and behind these were bushes, plants and trees including the most delightful Paulownia Tomentosa tree, of Portuguese extraction, which boasted a lilac trumpet shaped flower. Its branches wept down over the east corner. There was a certain air of the Secret Garden attached to this space because so few people knew of its existence, or were blind to its charms. I wasn't very keen to share the secret, a selfish emotion I know, but one of its many faceted attractions was the solitude and silence. A sylvan sense of nature embraced you. Reminders of the countryside's charm pervaded and helped provide an equilibrium to my mind that my carcass was incapable of supplying.

Without such respite the immediate surrounds of the ward forced melancholia on all of us and confronted you with debate about the one truly philosophical problem. You know…that of suicide, judging whether life is or is not worth living. To answer this would be to answer the fundamental question of philosophy, and I can tell you without equivocation that the answer is yes.

For I was far from alone, and surrounded by too many strident examples of optimism to dwell too long in such torpid isolation, to toy with the no word. Besides, Suzi would never have given me permission.

Amidst the sadness of ill health there are people who work every day helping the nurses to get people better. Auxiliary Care Helpers have a humour which is deprecatory.

Their preparedness to do difficult, awkward and menial tasks made me realise just how lucky I was to have spent so much time working in the comfort blanket of palatial hotels.

My career had suitably servile beginnings, but I had grown up through the ranks to become an owner and operator of hotels with the sort of character, facilities and style that customers dreamt of coming to stay at. This allowed me to live like a millionaire, bypassing the need to become one!

If you need a diet coke at 2 a.m. just dial room service.

What bitter irony that I should have devoted so much time catering for generally self-obsessed people to whom staying in posh hotels became a right, putting their happiness ahead of mine. Because now the role was wholly reversed and I, the selfish customer didn't just need coke at 2 am… I needed to receive dedication in return, from anyone who would pay attention.

How I rejoiced when Rupert from bed 6, one fine morning strode across the ward to the reception desk dragging his catheter trolley behind him and announced, 'I wish to check out, please prepare the bill and have the car brought to the front.' They tranquillised him and put him back to bed. He died the next day. The bill remained unpaid in one way but at too high a price in another.

The nurses, it increasingly appeared, dished out the drugs while the care workers washed me, carried me, dressed me, fed me, nurtured me and never made me feel as though I was asking too much. For their collective strength and individual humility I shall always be grateful. Of course there were stars but all were very special people.

There is an expression which now pervades the NHS which is supposed to sum up a perceived malaise. Apparently present-day nurses have become 'too posh to wash', leaving the lion's share of the duties to the care workers who are in theory the least trained and qualified members of the workforce. This may have been true, but what I did undoubtedly perceive was that whenever the teams worked together as one unit, with purpose, the patients got looked after more quickly, the general mood was lighter and there always seemed to be time to spare. When those members of the brigade who were more obsessed with hierarchy took charge, anarchy broke out in the ranks, less work got done, patients were more at risk and a sense of unrest hung uneasily in the air.

Behind most major illnesses today there are a number of charities, trusts and supporting bodies.

It was still a surprise though to find out that such a little known ailment as mine should possess such a wide ranging level of help.

The GBS association have set up a voluntary support group and added a green tortoise to their logo. It was almost entirely comprised of volunteers who have past experience of the illness. I was fortunate to come under the guiding wing of John Beaven.

A local journalist who had fallen prey to the syndrome some five years previously, John had made a full recovery save some tingling in his feet. Armed with the most considerate manner he came to see me once a week, never overstaying his welcome and always prepared with advice appropriate to the next stage of my recovery. The pastoral care that he offered was an elixir.

It was a privilege to have known him and a permanent bond was burned deep inside. That he should call from his annual holiday in France to check on my welfare spoke volumes for the quality of the man.

To our delight and surprise we realised that our parallel lives had crossed before. Some 20 years previously I had sat next to his wife for dinner in the Cotswolds. We both shared a passion for Bath Rugby Club's many triumphs (and escalating list of inglorious moments) and one of my oldest pals had worked with him at the same desk for the major local paper for 5 years.

He had covered all sports in the winter and one in particular from April to September... yes... with spring came cricket.

The local ground was adjacent to the hospital. Known as the Lansdown cricket club, this was the pitch on which the great Sir Vivian Richards first made his debut in England. It was also the area on which helicopters landed with accident and emergency cases flown in from the surrounding counties. In Canterbury, the home of Kent County cricket club, an antique oak tree stood unbowed for centuries within the boundary of the ground. The white rope which marked out the edge travelled happily around the perimeter until it met this old tree and was brought in around the front of it. If your stroke hits the tree stump before hitting the ground you score a six. Such idiosyncrasies should be preserved in life and sport lest the world become like the high streets of every market town in England: identical!

Admittedly this cricket pitch didn't have quite the same level of history or romance attached to it, but it certainly had its protocol. No matter how delicately poised the outcome of the match taking place on the pitch was, play had to be interrupted the moment the players or umpire first heard the whir of any helicopter rotor blades. If the bowler had started his run-up then the delivery was to be completed but the rest of the over was suspended while the players retired to the clubhouse.

Replete in its indigo blue livery the ambulance helicopter would draw near, scattering spectators in its wake. The emergency team rushed out with their stretcher trolleys and drew as close to the circumference of the rotating blades span as they dared. It was quite a spectacle. Critical cases from all over Gloucestershire, Somerset, Wiltshire, Devon and Dorset were regularly rushed expeditiously into the womb of the intensive care unit to receive treatment and medicine instantly.

Once the helicopter had set off for its next mission and a prudent interval had been allowed to pass, then play would resume just as tenaciously as before. The quality of games varied enormously.

Sometimes an ex-England standard opening bowler would open the attack, and at other times the novice 11-year-old, without hand to eye co-ordination, would close it, all too quickly, why, even the ladies got in on the act.

Strapped into and pushed out on my wheelchair we would potter along the corridors away from the ward, to while away 30 minutes watching matches of all standards, graduating to a crafty 1/2 pint of beer from the white timbered clubhouse, as my confidence grew. My arms still did not work, but the pain was shifting from my body, millimetre by millimetre. The spine, which had been in the most intense pain, had recovered some feeling and some strength. My arms and legs remained unimpressed at the prospect of doing any work. The hands never stopped hurting in the most aggressive fashion. However once you become used to the pain you just accept it as part of your daily life.

The sense of helplessness was still all-engulfing. Apart from being able to move my head from side to side and open and close my mouth and eyes, there was little other movement I could initiate or congruous sound I could truly project. There were still too few reasons why anyone should want to talk to me.

Yet the most increasingly restorative medicine was beginning to come less often from what had been mainly one-way conversations. Now close to two-way, I 'chatted' with nurses, fielders at silly mid on, care workers, Suzi (always) and my family of philanthropic friends.

That springtime was an inspiration. It brought variety, it brought change of scene and it encouraged movement. Perfecting my standing to begin walking became the next objective. I had learned how to become upright, by being turned into position on a tilt table. The next frontier was the hydrotherapy pool, which helped my flexibility and enabled me to stand and take the faintest steps supported by water. It seemed so liberating to be in water. That was until my first meeting with Kirsten's breasts.

With great generosity, it seemed to me, she filled her swimming costume in the most ample way. Proportions became vital, although relative. At exactly five foot one she was 14 inches shorter than I, so there was no justifiable reason why my chin should be so inexorably attracted, by magnetic force, to her bosom.

But there my chin hovered, dipping and diving in one convulsion after the next as I struggled manfully to straighten my spine and stand to attention (in the non-biblical sense). I still maintain that I owe my ability to straighten up to these watery encounters.

Getting in and out of the pool was quite a performance. A crane was required which carried a specially adapted chair up and over the water in an arc before lowering any incumbent into the over-chlorinated depths. 36 degrees centigrade was a lovely temperature but essential for people like me with such poor circulation. For 20 blissful minutes or so I lurched around supported by two members of the physio team who knew how likely it was that I would capsize. I didn't let them down! Those early moments enabled me to practise my arctic roll over and over again, so that I could be ready to start advanced lessons in canoeing the very next day.

Shamelessly I was savouring these moments of being the centre of attention. The illusion was shattered when the first member of the 'Cripples' Fat Club', as they liked to introduce themselves, got into the water with me. She was followed by 12 more people over the next five minutes who entered the water in a variety of ungainly ways. Each had suffered some debilitating problem which had either resulted from an accident or neurological attack.

They looked as elegant as a daddy long legs after some recalcitrant child has sadistically pulled off several limbs. All were grotesquely overweight and once in the water proceeded to bob up and down keeping their efforts to burn off calories and improve their mobility to the absolute minimum. They just wanted to talk! It was like an aquatic coffee morning. The only part of their physique to receive any material exercise was their jawbone.

It was impossible not to get in their way but I wasn't interested in giving up my moments in the hydrotherapy pool. The sensation of warm water on the flesh and the opportunity to defy conventional gravity were so rewarding. Through this medium I was able to remind my muscles of the sort of work that they used to do. Their refresher course was of paramount importance. I would happily have spent all day, every day in that pool in spite of the fellow attendees. Sadly I was only able to visit twice a week, the control of visiting times was democratic and there were just as many other patients in equal need.

The status quo in my throat had begun to change.

I had been unable to project my voice for more weeks than I wanted to remember, resorting to exaggerated movements of the lips and inviting any listener to get as close to my face as they could bear to bring their gaze. It was extraordinarily frustrating for both parties.

Inevitably you end up repeating statements and requests several times, without understanding what it is in your delivery that the person trying to interpret cannot grasp. Some nurses seemed to have a special antenna which enabled them to tune in immediately, barely missing a word. Others might as well have been studying Esperanto.

Curiously the most attentive were the Spanish nursing staff. Out of an aggregate of 1200 full-time employees in the hospital, 108 of them were from Spain. Evidently their medical training system had created too many applicants for too few jobs. So their health authorities had gone into the export market and the United Kingdom were happy to oblige. They arrived with finely honed nursing skills and a mixed bag of 'wordsmithing' abilities.

The one first assigned to me was called Manuel, all the way from Barcelona! A handsome and charming, tall 21 year old who only needed to look at a girl for them to understand any language he chose.

Because they were so used to asking people to repeat themselves to help them improve their language, understanding me did not seem so difficult. After all I had to enunciate slowly and with great exaggeration to make myself understood. I must have reminded them of their early language tapes in which they tried to comprehend our fascination with 'The Rain In Spain Staying Mainly On The Plain'. The sinister rasping sound, which escaped my throat whenever I tried to speak, came from my need to exhale words rather than inhale them. It was extraordinarily stressful and tiring because the neck muscles were so reduced and my lung power was minimal.

Humans speak with remarkable laxness and imprecision, yet we manage to express ourselves with subtlety at breathtaking speed. In normal conversation we speak at around 300 syllables a minute. Forcing air up through the larynx or 'supralaryngeal vocal tract' then pursing our lips and flapping our tongue to shape the passing puff of air into a loosely differentiated series of plosives, fricatives and gutturals.

This emerges as a more or less continuous wall of sound. We Do Not Talk Like This, wetalklikethis!

It helps to picture a watercolour painting left out in the rain to remember just how our syllables, words and sentences all run together. Getting the words onto the painting page in the first place meant practice and patience, for voluble I was not, nor pleonastic.

Mellifluous, that was how I wanted to be, no matter how many duff paintings I made on the way.

For those stroke victims around me who had been struck down the right side of their bodies speech was a real difficulty. Learning how to use your second hand late on in life is difficult enough, but expressing yourself with severely or permanently compromised speech was something I could not comprehend, far less accept.

My body though, was learning new alternate ways in which to express itself, particularly through a recovering appetite. Was it magic, centrifugal force, or willpower that had kept me upright in the swimming pool? It certainly wasn't a balanced nutritional diet. The hospital offered a three-week rotating menu which never varied by season. There were all kinds of pies, fish pies, ocean pies, shepherds pie, pie from cottages, and 'Specialite du Maison' exhausted steak without any kidney pies. Even without the muscle wasting illness the lack of intellect in the planning of the National Health Service's menus meant my chances of recovery were severely compromised.

Continuing to serve food from a cook chill menu so mundane, so lacking in aspiration, so contemptible should have been a hanging offence. I had lost weight at a spectacular pace, dropping from 15 stone to 11 and a half and held out no prospect of gain with this pie in the sky diet.

Amidst all this ribald entertainment, occupying the mind to overcome such distractions became more important. So I tried to graduate from counting the panels in the ceiling, through trying to remember the names of all the staff, to listening to audiotapes. Ricky Tomlinson became my favourite as he told his life history from casual entertainer, through picket on lightning strike and a spell in prison, to his finest hour encouraging the nation to say 'My Arse' sitting in a big armchair in the classic British sitcom, the Royle Family. There was something sad, yet encouraging, about his Liverpool tones and something so wonderfully Scouse about his excuse that everything was always someone else's fault.

I had been trying to work out who was at fault in my own case. Admittedly, the previous year had been quite stressful, a deal had taken too long to complete, and certain projects had been slow to progress.

What had I done wrong? Who was to blame? Could I have done things differently?

Question, after endless question revolved around the bedside, but I couldn't come up with an answer. The purchase of London's premier club-cum-hotel Home House had been completed two weeks prior on the sixth of December.

It was a long and protracted process which had spread out over an entire year and placed a considerable strain on our team. The lawyers had a field day and we hit many points when giving up seemed the only sane option. I am delighted we didn't because the business is quite unique and has grown strongly since but the stress of chasing the deal was nothing so out of the ordinary that it should cause a collapse like mine single-handed.

There had seemed so much to do, the sense of excitement had been palpable, and at last it had become action stations. I had just turned 50. This, I had hoped, was to be a year of milk and honey. Then it vanished.

But I was the lucky one. I had a return ticket. Every other patient I met had a new level of compromise in their life and had only booked a single flight.

Motor neurone disease, cerebral palsy, ME and MS, meningitis, stroke, aneurysm these were the stock ingredients, but some folk were given cocktails!

How about septicaemia, major organ failure, heart surgery sprinkled with nutmeg and topped with a final burst of Guillain-Barre, for good measure. Oh, I nearly forgot, Mike Harvey a brother in arms from our college days, was in a coma for months as well....but more of our reunion later.

Whenever I started to feel sorry for myself I had to stop. It wasn't realistic to harbour petty jealousies when I was constantly surrounded by people who were so much worse off than me. My lifeline had always been and remained Hope. Hope that things would improve. Hope that there would be a next stage to life worth looking forward to. Hope that there might be a regime beyond faith and charity. It was these latter two ingredients that provided the only embrace to so many of my companions.

'He that is down needs fear no fall, he that is low needs fear no pride,' said Gabriel, my neighbour in bed no 4. They were the last words he spoke to me or anyone for that matter, as he never woke up afterwards.

In some cases the state of the visitors appeared even worse than that of the patients housed in the ward. One particular father had been battling with cancer for many years only to be struck down with a heart attack which hit him on the right side of his body. This left his mouth skewed at a funny angle and removed most of his speech faculty. His dutiful wife visited every day. So used to the hospital environment, after so many visits she was completely unfazed by the surroundings.

Their sons, though, were a mixed bag.

The eldest had been caught in a car accident which had broken many of his bones before the car burst into flames and set fire to most of his body. It was quite miraculous that he was alive and even more staggering that his spirit was still so contented. He matched this with a genuine concern for others and refusal to be broken. Looking in the mirror each day must have been a constant reminder of the agony and devastation that the accident had wrought.

The middle son had a scary form of gigantism which enlarged his bones in awkward places and for instance, made his hand span quite disproportionate to the rest of his frame.

His eyes popped out of his head like an insect as if attached on stalks.

The youngest son had inherited the good looks, the eye for the ball, the silver tongue and all the good genes going. With such a head start you would have expected him to be the Sampson of the family, taking the collective weight on his shoulders. Unfortunately there was an addictive side to his personality and he would invariably turn up to visit his father drunk as a lord. This did not stop dad sharing out his love equally among his boys. Although he was bound by the vows of silence his illness had imposed on him he still communicated his affection by gesture, lopsided smile and hearty laugh. This man had been in and out of hospital for years. His wife could barely remember the last time they had enjoyed life without such enduring obstacles marring their best endeavours. How I wished I had some special magical powers, to provide them with the alchemy which would re-programme and vivify their flawed destiny.

After all I had developed a soft drinks business making own label specials for Pret-A-Manger and other high street notables, ranging from elderflower, lime, grape, apple and spring water to lemon grass, schizandra, ginko and ecinachia... so blending things came easily to me. Or at least it used to. That was the old genial, gregarious me. Now I was an island, a Robinson Crusoe on Friday's day off, living in mental isolation in vituperative ignorance, unaware of my effect.

Thus I was not aware of the tragic figure that I presented to them. For all my sympathy stretching out across to that family they returned the affection with interest. In their eyes my story was every bit as woeful, in mine tears were forming.

I closed my eyes to hide them, hoping to drift off to sleep before the late shift clocked on. I did not succeed.

The ward teams worked in three eight-hour shifts which rotated through early, late and night. Most of the staff worked a combination of all three shifts, a few just worked for the day but the SAS storm troopers just did the nightshift.

These were the hardy souls, who balanced gloom and doom with a raucous sense of mischief. I gave them nicknames which they never knew. Blofeld was the first, a cheerful lad who lived on a farm by day, treated me like someone he could talk to but was wrapped up in his plans to get married on the seventh of the seventh month in 2007.

Could I help him find an Aston Martin to be the wedding car? Of course, I wanted to say, pass me my jacket, there's one in my coat pocket.

Yogi was inevitably a bear of a man, as wide as he was tall, the strength of one of the shire horses from animal farm and a surprisingly cerebral personality.

After Ricky Tomlinson I had turned to poetry for my easy listening. Yogi overheard "If" by Rudyard Kipling, and immediately turned the volume down so that he could recite the words directly to me.

Where it took three nurses to adjust my position, it took one tug of his strong arm to yank me back up the bed. His surfeit of strength gave me vicarious pleasure.

What energy I had left seemed just out of reach, it had exited at such speed, and hadn't left a forwarding address.

The jailer was an altogether different specimen. How she had become a nurse I shall never know. She had the perfect personality to work on the complaints desk at Easy Jet. Loud, vulgar, abusive and hungry she would skip her duties as quickly as possible so that she could open a can of Coke, and wade her way through the first of her night-time Indian or Chinese takeaways, belching with sapient delight. Each night you prayed that someone else would be allocated to look after you, but if you were unlucky then the best form of defence was attack. Somewhere inside this termagant must have been a caring soul but my goodness, how hard she fought to hide it.

I can still hear those keys jangling now.

Meantime back on the day shift, the person opposite me wanted a fag. Their lungs had collapsed, they were coughing up blood, and they had just had a heart attack.

This was a mere inconvenience which meant that their next cigarette had been delayed.

Outside the front of the hospital, relatives would puff away at the little white stick in their hands as if winning the lottery depended on the next drag.

Often they were accompanied by patients who would walk out in their fluffy slippers, pushing their intravenous drips on a chrome trolley beside them.

In subzero temperatures women, plumbed into their catheter bags, wrapped in hospital issue nightgowns would gather in a tribal ritual by the smokers' shelter and stand outside it no matter what amount of rain or snow was falling. They stayed outside because inside the shelter stank of stale cigarettes!

Not one of them was struck by the irony of this last point, nor, more importantly did they care what they were doing to their health; the tobacco addiction was in absolute control.

Maybe, just maybe, there is a link between our health and our behaviour.

I had already decided that there must be, so sought out any assistance I could find to get me better. In addition to helping me relearn the art of standing in the pool a whole galaxy of implements and devices were incorporated into my daily routine. At night my feet would be placed into plaster casts to reduce the effect of the foot drop.

These casts were made on-site, to order, and rebuilt every three weeks to encourage the rake of my feet to return to a position close to a 90 degree angle to my shin. By day splints were placed around my ankles and hamstrings to help me stand and lift my feet. Without them I could have hit the ski slopes and hurtled down a black run in Courcheval. Every session with the physios' was designed to get me comfortable to sit up, then stand, then walk. To get from a sitting position on the edge of the bed and into a wheelchair the team took me to the gym and upgraded me to a banana board. As the name implies this piece of wood is shaped in a curved L. Half of it is shoved underneath one of your buttocks, on the side of the bed, leaving the other half to project out over the wheelchair. One of the armrests on the chair is removed allowing you to slide across the board and into the seat. It is much easier said than done and requires considerable focus from the physios and a series of bunny hops from the patients.

The tasks sound so simple and mundane but to me they were incredibly difficult.

Preparing for each hop, which might at best move me a couple of inches to one side, required the same focus and effort as running down the track at an Olympic pole vaulting contest.

My arms still appeared as though they had nothing to give and my fingers hurt like hell. The occupational therapy team led by the lithe and deceptively strong Shona massaged my hands every day.

You needed a microscope to see any improvement but that didn't stop us looking. The manipulation of my hands provided temporary relief and miraculously uncovered the tiniest movements. The little finger on my left-hand could wiggle from side to side. Hallelujah day! It couldn't go up or down or turn but it was a start. The middle finger of my right hand started to straighten.

The muscle had eroded completely, leaving loose flesh in all its wasted glory hanging between each digit. Without prompting, these skeleton hands would curl inwards forming a curious and sinister claw like shape. Hand splints were supplied to be worn at night and whenever resting by day. This was to help the wrist, palm and fingers rediscover a more normal position, albeit in an artificial habitat.

There was nothing spectacular to report about this series of incremental steps which proffered no more than marginal improvement. It was a slog!

Fortunately they possessed a technologically advanced piece of machinery which enabled a cumulative effect to build up from a very meagre beginning. By embracing it I was able to accelerate the pace of my recovery but also the volume of muscle repetitions which I could achieve in any one day without my legs giving up on me completely.

This wondrous battery-powered portable contraption was introduced to assist my attempts to complete what to you is the easiest task but to me was mission impossible namely to stand up. Specious in a shocking livery of purple, yellow and grey the Arjo Encore became my 'must have' travel companion.

Picture a fork lift truck in miniature where the forks are reversed in underneath the feet of the operator.

I would sit on the edge of the bed as the machine was wheeled backwards towards me. My feet would be placed on to plinths as a belt was wrapped around my middle and held in place by a rigging system clearly designed by a yacht builder.

It brought back memories of my first attempts at learning how to water ski. My hands were strapped on to two metal levers which rose upwards as the belt pulled me inexorably towards the main shaft of the machine, leaving me with no option but to achieve a standing to attention pose. The theory was fine, the training manual was lucid but the practice was very different.

The levers hauled my arms up alright. The belt dug into my buttocks to shift my frame, and the machinery hauled the legs up into the air.

So far so good, except for my right ankle which turned outwards in the process taking all of my weight through it once I was fully upright. Without the reflexes to shift my weight to my left side I could only signal my reaction by exhaling belly grunts of displeasure. These were not cries of pain, it was worse than that. I sounded like a sea lion berating a mate. You might think I was making a fuss but I couldn't stand properly on my right leg again for three weeks, in spite of cold compresses, regular physiotherapy and acupuncture.

If it was this difficult for me goodness knows how someone like Douglas Bader had been able to cope. If he could learn to walk again without his own legs and start to play golf to a decent standard then I wasn't going to let this be anything other than a minor setback.

The good news was that the muscle memory loss was so close to absolute that one day I might relearn golf without retaining all those unreliable habits I had added to my haphazard game over too many years.

So let's have some dramatic fairway striding exercises, to get in the mood.

Cometh the hour cometh the harness!

This system was dreamt up by the head physio who without realising it had become my hero. Kirsten had the gift of being able to make you do things your body didn't want to do, more often than you ever believed possible and to repeat the exercise the next day and somehow make it pleasurable. Like a young child's first pair of dungarees the harness was wrapped around my chest and groin, it was attached to a track in the ceiling in the vacant ward next door.

Slowly the harness, and therefore I, was winched upwards from my wheelchair toward the ceiling until my legs were straight. I could raise my left leg an inch or so, just enough to begin the process of walking.

The right leg did not want to join in however and trailed behind, like Quasimodo's haunches. I had a tall frame, with wheels on, in front of me on which to rest my arms, known as the pulpit.

I was too out of breath in seconds to deliver a sermon but with a great deal of coaxing I managed ten paces and collapsed quite exhausted. The following day we managed 12 paces and so the process went on.

'Kick out like an ostrich!' came the instruction.

Apparently ostriches splay their feet when they walk. This made me want to sing. So there we were, two physio instructors and I, lurching across the floor with my left foot splayed, Quasimodo's right dragging behind... singing 'Springtime for Hitler and Germany', yes The Producers had arrived all the way from Broadway. Admittedly we didn't manage the goose step on day one but most mornings brought some marginal improvement and after a month or so I was ready for the pulpit without the harness. My groin was in ecstasy.

Weeks of the 'dungaree nether regions' had forced me to sing springtime in falsetto, now I could tackle baritone.

By putting pressure down through the elbows I was able to take some weight onto the pulpit to give my legs a chance of bearing the rest of me. I had some limited strength in my shoulders and the top of my triceps, none in my biceps or any part of my hand or forearm, but it was a start. Goodness knows how toddlers manage.

I don't remember it seeming such hard work when I was their age. An hour of this a day was all that I could manage. But my mind was active and my speech was starting to return, why there was even some level of timbre returning to my voice.

Now if I could just find a sympathetic patient with some of his wits about him, I could try to contribute a bit to a proper conversation.

Ian was 44 years old, on his second marriage with two young children and suffering from a congenital heart problem, which he shared with his three brothers. Once in the army he had served his time abroad before returning to set up his own business.

He had accepted the deck of cards that life had dealt him and found aces and kings where others could only see the two of clubs.

His business had thrived, then one day quite unannounced he fell over. This was the first sign of the heart problem that was to dog him for years to come.

He seemed to take pleasure from talking to me in his broad Scottish brogue; I was an eager listener. He explained how he had lost the business, the marriage, the first wife and the fancy motorcar when his health gave way. He believed he was stronger for the experience and showed an inner warmth and calm that belied the parlous state of the left side of his frame. When on active military duty he had spent many hours in the company of the Ghurkhas whose attitude to possessions and the pursuit of material things refreshed him.

One particular orderly had impressed him when outlining his plans to buy a scooter. The Ghurkha was saving money as fast as he could to buy a scooter to take back to the village. But the scooter was not for him. Even though he was buying it, he did not need to own it. It was his gift to his village high up in the mountains.

The story invigorated me.

It set me thinking about the chase for the Yankee dollar and suddenly I became very conscious of the profit and loss account that is our life. If my own illness proved anything it was that we should be very careful how we spend whatever years we have. People can tell you but it takes a loss to comprehend value. Do not waste a moment as time is such a precious resource, and of course the only certainty in life is a reasonable probability.

Ian passed me an Everton toffee. It looked so appealing in its black and white livery. That toffee spent the night on the table next to my bed, complete in its clear wrapper.

The following day he noticed that it lay untouched and asked me why. Then he realised I couldn't use my hands to get the wrapper off let alone put the sweet in my mouth... We giggled at the absurdity of this scrimmage.

The following day he went back home, the hospital having said there was nothing more they could do for him except wait for the next downturn in his health. What a way to pass the days, waiting for the next relapse. His parting gift to me was another mint, with the words 'you will know when you are getting better because you'll be able to eat that sweet without any help.'

I felt introspective after he had gone.

Even though I couldn't project my voice very far I could at least make myself understood by now. Every day the strength of my breathing was measured on a puff machine to assess how much air I could exhale. The pitch was still soft and rather feminine and I favoured short sentences lest I run out of steam midway. I had reached the stage where I wanted answers to many questions about my prospects and the future. The matter which did not rest easy with me was the sense of injustice. I didn't have a foolish diet, I had never smoked cigarettes, I drank alcohol occasionally but rarely to excess and the closest I had ever come to taking drugs was a Fisherman's Friend.

I had been very fortunate to avoid hospitals, save for the birth of my children, for most of my adult life. Admittedly middle-age had crept up on me. You can tell when the hair from your nostrils grows more quickly than that on top of your head and your eyebrows start to give Denis Healey a run for his money if left unchecked.

Research into GBS was adamant that the illness was not stress-related, yet I had started to suffer compromises to my condition in the immediately preceding years which suggested that stress had started to become a factor. I didn't believe in stress, I thought it was one of those 1990's expressions which had carried on into the new millennium but which should have been permanently consigned to a dusty library shelf; a bit like crop circles, crystals, the word *holistic* and Chris de Burgh.

Maybe I should have studied my tea leaves more carefully. The omens were harbingering away if only I had seen them. The more I thought about it the more I realised the last few years had been relatively poor ones in terms of my physical condition. A series of events had combined against my welfare. Like most men who refuse to read a map when they desperately need directions I had failed to spot the signs, far less interpret them and do anything about it.

An outrageously gifted trompe l'oeil artist who could paint any flat surface and kid you it was 3D had taken hold of my hand the previous summer. He studied my palm and began to stumble over his words. He had bad news and needed to compose himself. 'I've got trouble with your life line, it just sort of stops over here and then starts again over there. It's almost as though you have two lives, I won't go on if this is upsetting you.'

'Jez, you old fraud,' I'd said. 'Just get on with it.'

He swallowed and proceeded to tell me things about my life history he could not possibly have known before warning me that my second life line started up again after a big gap, a schism of epic proportions. He told me to learn from the past and hoped

I wasn't about to have a dreadful accident. I thought no more of that conversation until now.

So what could history teach me? Well there was big Willie for a kick off...

Willie John McBride was arguably one of the most ferocious and feared rugby players that the British Isles has ever exported on a Lions tour; Quite the gentleman off the pitch and an archetypal animal on it. When asked to describe his most difficult opponent he cited his gallbladder. The pain prior to its removal was the most malicious he had ever experienced. This we had in common.

I too had felt that red hot poker stabbing away inside my stomach, to be followed by the sweet briar of release, when a skilled surgeon whipped out the offending gallstones, three years prior.

When I had woken from the general anaesthetic and all was done, my children showed me the resultant trophy.

Two gallstones the size of liar dice in a specimen jar, which smelt like a used packet of pork scratchings. Hard and pitted like golf balls they glared at me, defiant to the last. My eldest boy announced that he planned to exhibit them to his classmates, so away they flew, but via the silver specialist who presented me with a fine pair of cuff links, trapping the gall inside their metal coffin. Revenge was indeed a dish best served cold! Although not before every lad in his class had seen the uncut version first.

Evidently the operation had put my system through trauma and there was a 50-50 chance that psoriasis would hit my skin approximately six months later if I had a history of this illness in my family, which of course I did. Right on cue my flesh started to bubble and burst with an excess of skin production matching symmetrically down my body. Red and angry by sight, it came aboard 2 by 2, at the back of my elbows, side of my calves and around the knees in particular. Pungent smells abounded as all sorts of potions, remedies and creams were applied to little avail over the ensuing months.

Time for the UVB light treatment!

This was to be paid for by my private health insurance scheme, but administered by the national health hospital. The nurse instructed me to take off my clothes behind the screen and put on a pair of goggles. 'Now I want you to go and stand inside that cabinet over there, which has the vertical light tubes inside it. When I have closed it and turned the light on lift up your left knee and right elbow to point at the light source, and then alternate.'

'Let me get this straight, you want me stark naked wearing a pair of goggles inside an upright coffin doing a Morris dance?'

'Yes, that about sums it up,' she replied. 'Oh, there is just one other thing. We do recommend that you protect your genitalia.'

'Pray tell me how in all its infinite wisdom does the NHS propose to protect my genitals for me?'

'We recommend a black sock.'

My skin cleared up in no time at all. I really can't decide whether it was down to the special light treatment or the stress relieving guffaws that poured out of me each time I put that sock on. Marked 'Large' of course!

If you are a gambling man you will appreciate the odds. 50-50 seems pretty fair if you are placing even money. But a 1 in 14 chance of the psoriasis triggering psoriatic arthritis made this bet a rank outsider. Sure enough, it romped home about three months later. Pins and needles in my index fingers and thumbs, lack of grip and oblique sensations, together with a swelling in my right knee which required regular draining, became my new companions.

Now gambling with money is one thing but gambling with your health was not something I wanted to do. I hadn't reckoned on my personal bookmaker deciding to raise the stakes still further with his very own GBS accumulator. This time the odds were even more spectacular at 100,000 to one. Who needs the lottery? The tingling in my fingertips which had arrived with the arthritis was a gentle introduction to the virulence of the assault on my nerve endings which had built up in such a short space of time once my immune system had started to crash out of control.

The last few years had offered an insight into the perils of ill health, but nothing more. I had not become used to being under the weather.

For the first time in my life I had met my match, this was the point where I had literally run out of steam, leaving me inert and grateful for anything which reminded my tired frame of movement and activity. I would never dismiss my health, underestimate the importance of diet or postpone exercise again. The lesson had been well and truly learnt, here in my new necropolitic home where the walls were made of perdition, the roof smelt so fusty and the windows offered such a mawkish view.

"I feel so awful that I did not take the time to find out how it really felt for members of my family and friends to be when they were unwell, lying in pain in hospital before they died... I won't make that mistake again" - Renny Dindyal, 'Brooklyn Tribune'

*** *** ***

"I feel as though I have known Sheppard for years, as though he has always been such a good mate, kind and generous... yet that slightly anarchic uncle I never really, really understood" - Amanda Ashley, 'Portland Times'

*** *** ***

"Despite (or perhaps because of) the tragedy of his situation, the way he writes is just a hoot !!!" - Victor Ubogu, ex-England Rugby International

CHAPTER FOUR
HOW TO WIN FRIENDS AND INFLUENCE PEOPLE

Behind the paid workforce there was an army of unpaid volunteers. Known as the friends of the hospital, they frequently gave up time to serve in the coffee shops, man the mobile library and even bring their pet dogs round for companionship.

Each morning about 11am one of these volunteers would come to dish out the tea from the three-wheeled trolley (it used to have four, until one broke off). The faces became familiar as did my response, a beaker of tea with a straw please. Generally the volunteers had their favourite days, so did I. Longing for Tuesdays. This was the day when I got my digestive biscuits and cup of char from a "Titled Tea Lady". Lady Farquhar had obviously been a stunner in her day and could have told me that my head was on fire and still made me smile, so serene was her countenance. Always immaculately presented and blessed with a still beautiful face, she made a fabulous brew and dished out the biccies with élan. Sometimes I even got a piece of cherry cake.

She invited me to come and visit her little garden when I was finally released from hospital and fully well. This was the most amatory thing to happen to me since I was admitted to the hospital. I had been transported into a DH Lawrence novel and there I was going into the field and bringing back the harvest, straight out of the passionate bit in The Rainbow. Or could I be Mr Darcy, just for a while, as the steam comes off my open shirt and breeches straight after swimming through the lake?

Hoping for a little frisson with a 68-year-old, albeit very well groomed, pensioner may not be your idea of romantic idealism. But it certainly made the chocolate bourbons taste a bit spicier.

My emotions will, I am sure, remain unrequited but she had lovely ankles and her idea of a little garden was 40 acres, Suzi knowingly approved of the weekly twinkle in my eye.

As a schoolboy I sat next to a rotund asthmatic called John Isherwood. We had been inseparable in class, always sitting next to each other, always getting into mischief and always sticking pencils into each other's ears.

You know that sketch where the schoolmaster comes into the classroom, while all the boys try to stifle their giggles, and in slow motion the water filled fire bucket, impossibly propped over the half open door, crashes onto the master's head soaking him down to his shoes... all the funnier because he cannot see the humorous side?

Well, the whole of John's attitude to school was like that, and he never got caught.

I did!

Yes, in John's company I had always been snatching defeat from the jaws of victory, playing Stan Laurel to his Oliver Hardy. And there he was at my bedside in this hospital making me feel nervous. What possible reckless skulduggery could a horizontal paralytic and a by now very eminent and reputable barrister get up to in a hospital? John saw it as his duty to visit me regularly, abuse my fragile confidence, barrel me out of the ward in a wheelchair, regale me with side splitting stories, drink my squash and eat my grapes, ignoring my cries of pain and anyone foolish enough to get in our way. I loved him for it.

Another old school friend turned up to see me in hospital by accident. His life had crossed the Rubicon of public consumption along the way, since the last time we had met when going to see the first showing of the film Papillon with Dustin Hoffman and Steve McQueen, 32 years previously. I had kept abreast of his progress in the doctoring field principally by sitting next to the food writer for the Financial Times at dinner who, it transpired, had been suffering from Crohns disease. A rotting of the stomach is hardly the most conducive passenger to assist you in writing about food, but that was how he had met my old mucker. Dr

Andrew Wakefield spent many years trying to decipher what was going on inside people's bellies. He became notorious on a global scale when he moved out of his original sphere of expertise and started to publish his views on the link between triple vaccines and autism.

Vilified by the health profession in this country he had to move to Austin in Texas to earn a living.

He remains firmly in the public eye through the many television and newspaper articles which chronicle his perceived shortcomings as the row over MMR continues to rage. That didn't stop him being my mate, though, or his friendship with the desperate soul who was procumbent two beds away from me in the same ward.

Formerly the life and soul of every party, Gerry had suffered a massive stroke and was unable to speak, consume food by mouth or see very well. He had many, many friends, all hearty folk who stayed for minutes, but no family to stay for hours; most of the time he cut a particularly lonely figure. His ability to communicate was as reduced as his number of opportunities to talk to true friends, or chances of recovery.

Dr Andy implored me to take good care of Gerry, which I attempted to do but with limited success, except when we could find a willing interpreter to translate our best efforts at conveying messages. None of his friends stayed for long, they found conversation as difficult with him as I did, but in truth they had only been his friends when he was buying the last drinks at the bar.

I had been amazed and shocked by the number of visitors who came to see me; my feelings bordered on embarrassment. Some I had barely known for a few weeks, others I had known since childhood.

For a couple of school chums would have matched my expectations, instead my former headmaster, best pal, next best pal all the way from Australia, more next best pals in descending order, boys I had been form prefect to, games master, chairman of the Board of Governors, chairman of the old boys association and countless others made a pilgrimage to my bedside. Then came the college buddies, the work colleagues, business associates, neighbours, aunts, uncles, nephews, past employees; friends from America, Wales, Scotland, Ireland, and France, even Essex but don't worry it's only the one friend.

Some 15 years previously an exact contemporary of mine from school had been struck down by an illness from the Guillain-Barre family. Known as CIDP it paralysed Roger down the right-hand side in a way which confused the local health authorities. Far rarer than GBS, it was beyond the scope of the regional team. Off he went to London for plasma exchange but it wasn't identified or treated swiftly.

So although he made some good level of recovery his decline was not arrested sufficiently quickly to bounce back fully.

Roger breezed into the ward armed with a bottle of Guinness and a wide smile. Introducing himself as 'your friendly neighbourhood cripple' he began to set out in painstaking detail the many trials and tribulations that had hit him. Since the illness had first taken hold, his marriage and his business had fallen to bits and he struck rock bottom when depression wrapped itself around him. An engineer by vocation he adapted his life to his new-found status and embraced life with the one good hand left active. He fought off the depression, came to realise that he would never fully shake off the ravages of the CIDP, nursed his children through school and on to Oxbridge, opened his own garage, met a new girlfriend and made light of his disability. Never one to court pity, Roger's lack of regret and deflection of sadness provided a great tonic. If he could get through such a seismic attack on a similar level to the one that I had experienced than I really had no excuse to rest on my laurels.

Should you ever have the misfortune to be in the trenches fighting an old-fashioned war, Roger is absolutely the one bloke you want alongside. Not to fight the enemy, he would be as much use as a chocolate fireguard.

But to proffer courage, physical support with his left hand, handy tips about car maintenance or bizarre facts about the mortality rates of travelling circuses in Venezuela. His whimsical take on life would gladden the soul and he would help you pass the time admirably. Crucially you would never need to mention the enemy.

It wasn't just friends though, or creditors, even my bank manager dropped in. Indeed I had just offered the opinion that GBS was an illness that I would not wish upon my worst enemy when at that very moment a missive appeared offering great sympathy from that very worst enemy himself. Apparently he had contacted my office offering to come and see me. With deftness of thought they had suggested that a card would suffice.

They didn't want a visit from him to kill me off completely.

Of course rumours of my Huckleberry death had circulated, but these were greatly exaggerated!

In the case of young Daniel no exaggeration was necessary.

He had just been brought into the ward so comatose that it was very difficult to tell whether he was dead or alive.

A year to the very day after his best pal had been killed with meningitis the same illness had hit him and hit him hard too.

The pace of his decline had been breathtaking, one moment enjoying life to the full, the next battling for his existence in the intensive care unit. He lay in a coma for three days before drifting back in and out of consciousness. In addition to the paralysing effect on his arms and legs it had affected his eyesight. He put on a brave face for all the doting family members who showed him such vigilant and constant support. Then burst into floods of tears as soon as they had gone. Amidst all the many words of encouragement he knew that his chance of recovering his sight was slim in the extreme, he could hear all the words of praise from fellow patients in the ward but it was weeks before he could put faces to the voices. At the age of 24 he had once understood that his world included oysters, now the pearls had gone and life was just a swine.

His bedside was littered with an avalanche of unsuitable food. He could have sponsored Coronation Street with the amount of chocolate in his possession and unsurprisingly was managing to put on weight while the rest of us were losing pounds for fun.

Every day his friends and family would visit in relentless waves, washing over his bedside and regaling him with the same ubiquitous welcome, the expression 'all right' was invariably used. How I longed for a 'hello, how are you' or even a 'hiya', just to break up the monotony. After all, it's not as though we don't have plenty of greeting phrases already in use to choose from: 'Avast there, me hearties'...'watcher,'...'hey,'...or my favourite...'oi, oi saveloy' which is doing rather well thanks to one protagonist in Chipping Norton.

Perhaps if the use of 'all right' had received greater inflection or variation in semantic emphasis I would not have objected so strongly to this demonstrable lack of imagination.

Daniel was making a sterling recovery due in large part to the warmth and union of his family. In fact he started to improve so much on a daily basis that he seemed to be in competition with his immediate neighbour Bill.

Young William at the age of 64 had decided to take a marginally early retirement, and just gone off on a cruise with his wife when he experienced the first aneurysm in his brain.

He was airlifted off and brought straight to the hospital where it was clear to all that he was in a very distressed state, stuffed full of morphine and hallucinating wildly. Yet after four days he started to show definite signs of improvement. From an unequal start he and Daniel were going head-to-head in a competition to see who could make the most dramatic recovery to full health.

No sooner would one demonstrate that he could walk down the corridor with the Zimmer frame than the other would discard the frame and graduate to sticks. Even though Daniel was still struggling to see he was determined to make his cry for freedom a vigorous one.

I became very fond of them both. After all, I was their audience, I had been spending months as a spectator of life unable to participate in any meaningful way. Observation had become my speciality, it was the one thing I could do really well. The world was still spinning round outside and I had no choice but to become busy doing nothing. Reminding me of a line I once had to perform on stage in strictly amateur theatre.

'Players sir! I look upon them as no better than creatures set on tables and joint stools to make faces and produce laughter, like dancing dogs.'

Armed with this medieval quote I would set off each day, almost always with the indefatigable Suzi, to circumnavigate the globe in search of a suitable table, or at best the canteen and the friends of the hospital coffee shop in its fucshia pink-liveried majesty.

Seeking out hidden treasures like a stolen slurp of tea from a china cup and a nibble on a digestive tiffin, while watching the unwashed, the unwell and the unwilling do their dog dances on tables and stools nearby.

Watching other people doing things that were denied to me was a strange sensation. When you are able-bodied, tasks like climbing stairs, walking or cutting your own food do not register as liberating pastimes.

To me they appeared so pleasurable, so divine, what a thrill it must be to be able to take part in life, be active, perform tasks without having to summon the stamina or someone else to do it for you.

My horizons stretched to getting into a wheelchair to taste the sunshine and watch these different types of theatre.

Still kidnapped inside my own body being taken for a push in a wheelchair was a genuine treat. The fact that I could sustain a period of time sitting upright in such a chair was terrific progress in itself. More theatre came from trips to the duck pond, touring the on-site newsagent or best of all sitting under the auburn chestnut trees watching the sun go down over the village green, as dappled light picked out the ebony swallows darting, and the cotton white clouds soared over an azure sky before the wind put its shadow to bed at dusk.

Nick and Ali took me to see their son in a bit of theatre, never to be repeated but scored in my mind's eye forever. Young copper-haired Calum was attending his very first cricket school. He had never played before and competitive dad was determined that his son would one day open the innings for England. Marching to the crease and brandishing his bat the wrong way around Calum did not make the most auspicious start.

He missed the first three deliveries bowled at him. At best his father's smile could be described as rueful.

The exhortation 'just hit it, lad' certainly galvanised the seven-year-old who promptly set off with both arms straight out at his side as he bore down on the rest of the field firing bullets from the imaginary Spitfire that he had just become. After shooting everybody else in his own team and the opposition young copper knob sidled over to his perplexed dad answering the obvious 'what do you think you were doing?' question with a totally disarming 'being an aeroplane, silly.'

Back in the wards there was a similar sense of the surreal. I had been in the same bed for so many months that I was fast approaching veteran status. My good buddy Sundance had been allowed home twice, only to suffer relapses and find himself admitted back into the hospital again. His hopes crested when he was transferred to a specialist unit in Bristol.

There his condition was treated with a relatively innovative process called Campath and after putting his body through yet more steroids he returned for the third time to the ward for what was to be our final period in hospital together.

Daniel returned some weeks later, walking on one stick with some good measure of sight restored.

He was brandishing a copy of his local newspaper in which a special feature on the likelihood of his illness striking him in such a similar way to his former best friend was circled. He laid out the paper for us both to read, so proud of the honourable mention for Sundance and myself. Evidently it had been our hectoring and cajoling which had spurred him on.

Typical of the boy, he was always thinking of other people.

Although released from hospital at the same time as Bill, somehow you just knew that Daniel would not come back as a patient but that Bill had been allowed home too soon.

Sure enough he started a series of giddy spells coupled with loss of memory and balance, and was promptly readmitted. This time the news was not so encouraging, after further examination and scans he was advised that he had a tumour in the back of his brain. The choice was stark, risk having it removed in the faint hope of some measure of recovery with the very real prospect of death during the operation.

Or carry on for what was estimated to be at best three more years, with the tumour riding shotgun. He chose the latter, after the most tortuous period deliberating over such an impossible choice. The tears from his wife were hard enough to bear but when Bill himself broke down there was no choice. You had to join in. Nero himself could not have created more drama in the Coliseum no matter how many lions or Christians were put to the Gladiator's sword. There it was again and again staring me in the face, the most vivid pageant with more daily drama than you could possibly imagine or have the stomach for.

These distractions were there for a very real purpose; they forced me to observe and made me as proficient in absorption of detail as the finest blotting paper. You see the background reveals the true being of each man. If you do not possess the background, it makes man transparent. By so consistently studying man I was stocking up my library. Man's behaviour in adversity was becoming my specialist subject. They say man is made stronger by realising that the helping hand he needs is at the end of his own right arm. Now if I could only make contact with mine!

The gym was my playground where making contact with disenfranchised parts of the body was the sport. It was a quiet, clean space with primary colour signage and wide mechanical 'beds' in apple green or russet hues. Curtains offered notional privacy while one patient hid from another while struggling with their task at faltering hand or under tenuous foot. It was always cool and rather calm but with a pervading sense of fun thanks to an optimistic team.

When the physios had first tried to get me to sit on the edge of my bed they had explained how poor my posture was. I would only be able to recover my stability if I sat up in a more upright way. I was trying really hard to stretch my torso but impressed no one. They fetched a full-length mirror over to wheel in front of me some ten yards away. I recoiled in horror when I saw for the first time what I had become.

There it was incontrovertible evidence that I was now, in my stripped to the waist pose, the very picture of Methuselah with Buddha's belly bolted on the front.

Everything else was skeleton skinny except for the football stuffed inside my tummy, and a face which had aged a hundred and seventy years. I never looked in the mirror again. Therefore I had no real understanding of what messages my expression could be projecting to others around me. One of the great lessons of life they say is that the last thing you learn about yourself is your effect. In such a setting how could I effect change when change had so obviously had its effect on me.

I was still wrestling with this period of solitary confinement. Could I get parole for good behaviour, transfer to an open prison with more freedom of movement or at least redecorate my cell. The paint finish on the walls was so last year!

Adamant that I did not want any more visual confirmation of my debilitated state I concentrated on the bits of my body that I could see, the lower arms and hands, legs and feet. I sent out regular instruction to them, offered motivational team talks, conducted workshops and whispered sweet nothings to little avail. Movement was still so elusive. At best fleeting, at worst defiant, the motion in my limbs had been on walkabout for too long for the frustration not to surface. I started swearing like a trooper. Billy Connolly's autocue would have blanched at the volleys of invective which shot out at random, apparently beyond my control. I shocked myself but this didn't stop me from blaspheming every time I tried to rotate my arms only to see my wrists collapse in abject surrender. It was a pig of a time, what seemed like so much effort for so little reward.

Apparently I made some people happy which is an odd thing to consider when you are doing so much crying inside your hollow frame.

I didn't set out to do this but I confess that on the days when I did try 'miserable-ness' I couldn't really get on with it. So I tried being of good cheer instead. In spite of, or probably because of, the tragic theatre which was being played out by the most unwitting thespians in their agony and their despair.

To quench my thirst for more theatre I was consuming information at a rapacious rate. It filled the void, the gap left when visitors departed and the tear half formed as they turned into the corridor and away into the night air.

Talking books, CDs and DVDs abounded and on certain evenings I would find my entire bed transferred out of the ward and into the television lounge. Incapable of changing the channels or adjusting the volume my presence made it very difficult for anybody else to get into the room. So I lay there alone.

The very first film to appear was a new channel five programme called CSI New York. The beginning of the series was about a mad surgeon who captures young vulnerable women, plies them with drugs to induce a paralysis called 'locked in' syndrome, and leaves them in his basement unable to move or communicate. A veritable living death… hang on a minute…I don't want to watch this… it's a bit too close to home.

I can't change the channel, cry for help, or get up and walk out. The parallels between GBS and locked in syndrome are just too similar. I start sweating, my heart beat goes berserk. Try to close my eyes but can't stop the actors talking. Get me out of this room or better still out of this body now, please!

Nothing... locked in, locked on, just plain locked.

Then the late shift arrived and looked in on me exhausted, distraught and breathing heavily. I was so pleased to see them, so thankful that they represented escape. The shock of seeing a programme about a condition so similar to the effects of mine seemed obscene in such a sepulchral context.

Perhaps I'm not ready for the TV room just yet.

So through the day I tried to read newspapers. The logistics were tricky as I couldn't turn pages or prop a full size paper on my lap, so a typical sequence would go column five first, then two, and wait for a nurse to go by to refold the newspaper so I could study one and three.

Usually I couldn't find column four. Then I found the crossword page, this was manna from heaven, because it was enough to keep the brain occupied for some time without having to turn pages. Had I been able to fill in the answers that might have made me more competent; if you have no idea how difficult it is to complete the crossword trying to remember your previous answers and their effect on the next clue as you go, let me tell you it is tough.

Pretty soon this wasn't enough and the work of Mrs Su Doku took a grip.

I really enjoyed these number puzzles particularly as I had to get other people to fill in the answers for me. Remembering sequences of 15 or so numbers before hailing some poor unsuspecting visitor to use their pen and trying to hear what I was mouthing at them started out as a leap of faith. By practice and sheer cussedness I got the cobwebs out of my brain and the addiction began in earnest.

It taught me how concentration on one particular task can absorb you to such an extent that your mind can blank out other troubles.

In particular I was gaining some control over the awareness of the ever present pain in my body. There was no doubt that active distraction could relegate the perception of pain attacks considerably. Teaching my brain to gain control of things again rather than abdicate responsibility was just as vital in the recovery process as learning to walk or 'going out for a push'.

Some friends just try too hard to help. Desperate to entertain they want to bring a dynamic element to your life. They volunteer all sorts of activities which you are not ready for. Thus at a time when I had only just mastered sitting in a wheelchair for about half an hour without becoming uncomfortable David pitched up with a plan to take me out to lunch.

Forward planning was never his greatest strength and checking the dress code at the restaurant to establish whether pyjamas were an acceptable alternative to jacket and tie would not have entered his head. Nor the practical question of how to transport me from the hospital to the restaurant in the middle of town which was over 1 1/2 miles away. 'Where's the taxi?' I enquired to be told that he couldn't get one so he began the 'going out for a push' expedition. Refusing to accept the incline of the hills or the fact that he was 61 and my wheelchair had not passed its latest MOT we set off about as well prepared as a Richard Branson balloon flight.

To be fair the early part of the journey went quite well…

About the first hundred yards!

And then the cobblestones kicked in, this was not my idea of haemorrhoid heaven. By the time we got to the restaurant for lunch they were ready to serve afternoon tea. With much persuasion however they deigned to serve up bangers and mash which was delicious. My napkin thoroughly enjoyed the meal.

Dear old David had forgotten that I could not feed myself let alone get a glass of Merlot to my mouth.

The words party, tea and chimpanzee would be contained in the sentence best describing his valiant efforts to spoon feed me in the middle of a crowded restaurant in a high ceilinged, over chandeliered, Georgian pump room complete with Palm Court trio bashing out the Waltzes.

Then there was the journey back which felt twice as long and thrice as difficult for him, but not so bad for my bottom because I had managed to secure a leather bound copy of the wine list to rest my withered buttocks on. When we got back he had to have a lie down on my bed. It was almost nightfall.

Journeys were important, but most took place in my mind. It is amazing how many places you can go and visit in your head without preplanning, booking a flight, or worrying about all the things that will be waiting to be dealt with on your return. I had always fancied a visit to Novgorod in northwest Russia, close to Leningrad. Set just up from its own inland sea and cut in underneath the east of Finland it was one of the few, if not the only, port on a Russian river/coastline which could stay open throughout their supremely harsh winter.

The weather could freeze seas all along the Arctic facing edge of this fascinating country. The analogy was fairly obvious I suppose, as I was trying to keep my mind open while the rest of my body was frozen over.

The question I was most frequently asked was how do you cope with the boredom? The truthful answer was that I didn't experience it.

At no stage in the entire process of my incarceration did I ever once feel short of something to occupy my mind. What I did miss was the curious lightness of being. Moving a limb automatically, turning freely and without discomfort. Something as simple as being able to cross your legs appeared so sophisticated and clever.

The relative talking happily ten yards away has just rested his right elbow over his left arm and is waving his hand nonchalantly at no one in particular.

What a wonderful thing to be able to do, complex in the extreme, when you consider all the components that enable such fluidity of movement; yet so simple in the appearance of its execution.

I admit it, I was deeply jealous.

Obviously it helped to have visitors and things going on around you but if these were not available then a mental journey was easy to summon.

At the beginning most of the objects of my aspiration involved simple provision, for instance I can still vividly recall the size and shape of the chilled jug into which fresh orange juice, mandarin and passion fruit had been squeezed with ice cubes and a sprig of mint. How I craved to trace my fingers down the condensation on the outside of the jug, to be able to pick it up and pour out a long lasting glass of bright sunshine before sipping it and savouring it to my heart's content.

This fantasy about confection was eventually replaced by transports of delight, setting off to the sunniest climes, via Fantasia, Avalon and the Falkland Arms at Great Tew for a drop of snuff, a homemade gooseberry and nettle wine for the lady and a pint of Hook Norton in a straight glass for me.

Off to exotic places where you can drink rum punch all day and never feel drunk, the offshore breeze is always a gentle zephyr, the turquoise sea is so clear that you can see every kind of coral and exotic fish darting around your feet. Cut inland to a balmy river perch next the weeping willow, where the coxless pair glide by disturbing a cormorant or grebe on the plume of a rippling weir. Glance west to an idyllic finale to the perfect day where the sunsets are a brilliant reddish pink, monkeys run wild without bothering you and there isn't a dumped supermarket trolley in sight.

Call it Utopia, or Turks and Caicos, or just self-deceit it did not matter, because it allowed total freedom to travel around the world without visa, typhoid injection or leaving the bedside.

Set against this unashamed escapism was a routine which defined the shape and duration of each day.

When I first became aware of marginal improvement in my bodily functions I tried to measure my progress on a daily basis.

This did not work, principally because the changes were so tiny that it was virtually impossible to distinguish progress over what was such a relatively short period of time. So I changed currency and started dealing in new units of time.

The week became my Euro. No looking forward or back more than one week in either direction. I could calculate the percentages better in weeks. After all your nerves reconnect no faster than 1 mm per day and some parts of your body are more complicated than others so the reconnection slows.

Things also took a lot of practice. Nothing returns to you without supreme effort, a setback or two, and repeating the activity again and again.

CHAPTER FIVE
HELP! I NEED SOMEBODY

Most mornings I would be woken by the lovely Maggie. The first calling would be around 6:30 am; by seven everyone would be breakfasted and ready for a wash. Provided Maggie was on duty. Although she was fond of her sisters she lived in an all-male household with three sons. She didn't like working in the women's ward; apparently "ill men don't whinge as much". Getting me up for breakfast involved heaving my head forward and rearranging the pillows before the Weetabix was spooned into my mouth.

Tea was allowed to cool in a plastic beaker before I was invited to sip it while one of the staff sat holding the beaker for me. The only way I could help in a meaningful fashion was to tilt my head to one side.

In contrast with the rigidity of breakfast service you could be washed at any point between 7am and midday depending on who was in charge of the unit, who was in a good mood that day, how poorly the other patients were, but most importantly whether Maggie was on duty. She managed to make the work of three members of staff look grossly inefficient when set against the organised and determined way she set about looking after her men.

She also understood football's offside rule and could talk with authority about the fortunes, transfers and playing formation of most of the premiership teams. Possessing many meaningful insights into typical girl's talk like whether a 4-5-1 was better than a 4-4-2.

I was intensely proud of her because she had a unique ability to mix extreme kindness and sensitivity about people's sensibilities with a no-nonsense, hard-working and efficient method. When she went home though her work was not yet done, for one of her grown-up sons had been challenging since birth and although able to hold down a job with limited responsibility still needed substantial nursing as soon as she got back to her house. No matter how much on the job training any person is given I can't believe it is possible to be taught the kind of caring skills that she possessed.

Washing each day had been confined to variations on the classic bed bath. Anything more than this would have involved twenty minutes of two nurses' attention to get me into a hoist, swivel me up and over the bed and drop me into a wheelchair. So after months of this work shy regime, Maggie decided I needed hosing down and off to the shower we went, having been lowered to perch on a mobile commode and wrapped in sheets like an extra in A Christmas Carol. The legs were so weak that they slipped off the foot rest and dragged along the floor but once we got to the watering hole what a felicitous pleasure it was to feel fresh H20, without chlorine, on my body again.

It was also time for changing clothes. The haberdashery of habiliments was about to open!

In the beginning I had found it difficult to wear pyjamas all the time because my body temperature was so volatile. Eventually this settled down as did the choice of colours for my attire. This was all very well but the mould needed to be broken, if only to re-educate my thoughts into believing that I could be human again. So a range of T-shirts, baggy trousers and loose tops was born.

There was no sartorial elegance about this move but it added an extra level of structure to the day and was one of the building blocks to repatriation.

Every day I would have at least one session of fulsome exercise, plus on most days there was an additional session with the occupational therapy team.

It is very easy to confuse physiotherapists with occupational therapists unless you study the respective blue and green uniforms thoroughly. The divide in ethos though, is easier to spot.

The physio team tended to concentrate on getting the bigger muscles moving and dealing with fundamental issues like walking and getting in and out of bed.

The occupational therapy crew, however, concerned themselves with turning positions of disadvantage around. How to grip a toothbrush, how to get a shirt on when you only have strength in one arm and how to return the ordinary moments of people's lives back to them. They taught me how to get a jumper over my head and shoulders unaided for as far as I could go, stretching the boundaries of expectation and result in turn until I had total mastery of the combination of skills needed to complete what to you is a facile task. It took three months just to get my limbs and enough momentum into the right places and at the right speed, to get close. Because I had no concept of grip improvisation and adaptation was vital. The middle of my body had started to recover sensation, not necessarily with strength, and from there the repatriation of the nervous system spread out in an ever expanding circle. The fingers and toes formed the perimeter at the very back of the queue. The pain began to ameliorate by getting worse in the part of the body which was about to get better. Thus for instance my shoulders went from a position of no movement, and excruciating pain when put into any new position, before becoming even more painful to touch and very, very cold.

Parts of me felt that they had been removed and placed in a deep freeze until a thaw set in. The pain found a new home further down the arm leaving the shoulder to wake up again; and lo and behold the faintest movement appeared. The triceps recovered relatively quickly in the upper part of my arm, months before any sign of life in my biceps. It was a similar story in the legs between back and front.

My thumb, on the right-hand had developed a serious inferiority complex. Bashful in the extreme this digit had decided to hide behind the four other fingers that he shared my hand with. We would try talking to him, tickling him, pulling, pushing and prodding him, all to no avail.

He had competitors though. Not provided by me but by three other GBS sufferers who arrived within a month of each other in the women's and then the men's ward.

The fey teenage girl was totally out of it, brimful of anger, depression and despair. Struck from the nose downwards with all facial inflection removed, it was impossible to elicit eye contact let alone conversation. She was frightened out of her wits. But her thumbs worked!

The two young guys never overlapped. Joe appeared first, troubled by aches in his hands and seized up through his trunk. For a musician losing your finger control is tantamount to disaster but he fought back quickly and returned to work within months. He could play the banjo and write his music again before I was able to leave the hospital. With a shock of dark brown hair and fulsome beard he could have auditioned for a musical Jesus if the mood had taken him but not before he had conquered every Deep Purple record he could find. Joe was cool, garrulous, naughty and jolly all at the same time. By being there he helped me to understand the GBS illness better, by leaving before me he set a wicked pace to catch up with.

Nathan took a bigger hit and became paralysed from the waist down, save some freezing in the face muscles.

An engaging sort, he kept cheerful and rebellious. On one evening we sloped off from the ward in search of adventure… Each evening a ritual took place in the main concourse of the hospital about 8pm.

It took three men two hours to stack tables and chairs from outside the coffee shop and place them to the side of the atrium.

One of them was deputed to operate the floor scrubber and polisher which was a mighty beast and extremely noisy. It is of course vital to smoke a cigarette through such a ceremony and in truth it was this part of the work which needed the greatest attention, time and focus.

If done really thoroughly, the clearing and cleaning could be stretched to a 20-minute job for one man but by introducing the 'homage to one's fag' part of the proceedings it was possible to add another hour and forty minutes.

Curiously a lot of this period would be spent outside the building where the men would gather to pace up and down often in a figure of eight pirouette.

The cigarette would always be held on the inside of the hand between thumb and forefinger. It would be passed from one man to the next like the baton of a relay running team. Intensity was etched across the glazed yet focused expressions of these working men determined to extract the maximum satisfaction from their 'drag' as if it was the last thing they would ever do on earth. Thanks to the ritual that they put into this performance they were able to add the correct level of worship, devotion, pomp and circumstance into what became a compelling ceremony.

And sometimes the floor actually looked clean afterwards!

One evening Peter and Jane came to see me replete with picnic basket and a battery of Tupperware. They wanted to take me out to dinner. So we headed for the atrium and spread out our wares on the one table that the men had yet to stack away. It was an absurd moment of surreal propriety, laced with a plenitude of over the top grub. There was Champagne, Gravadlax, Crayfish Roulade, Stinking Bishop Cheese and Fine Napery. To cap it all a candelabra was produced and the candles lit.

You half expected a band of itinerant Peruvian Pan Pipers to appear bashing out 'Guantanamera' before passing the hat round... (cash will do nicely, credit cards not accepted, of course).

Conversation started well but became more and more compromised as the floor scrubbing pantechnicon was marched up and down the increasingly adjacent floor. The taste buds were being tickled but it was not an aural sensation, the noise was too invasive. The offer of a solicitous packet of cigarettes did the trick though, as the men took off with this treasure, prompting the usual two-hour performance to extend to a record shattering two hours and 45 minutes, leaving us in peace.

Quite simply we were having fun. This was a commodity which had been in such sporadic supply since my admission to hospital that I felt quite drunk with the unbounded happiness of the occasion. You can keep tea at the Ritz from now on because I have dined at the most exclusive Captain's Table. The pendulum was starting to turn. The highlights of the day were starting to outweigh the lowlights. Not by volume, but by their effect.

Cumulatively there were starting to be more things to look forward to in a day than to dread. The aggregate of all the help, support, visitation and affection I was receiving was compounding nicely. The elixir of life itself was doing me good. Like a tree which has been through the winter without any sign of life within its branches, the shoots of recovery were starting to bloom.

Initially this was just in the lower branches and the highest points of the tree would have to wait, but the sap was definitely rising.

Getting set for bed had a certain routine attached to it as I needed a series of exercises to be completed on my limbs, Suzi would complete this ritual for me religiously, as her last act before setting off home, but left my teeth to the night staff occasionally. Changing clothes and having the teeth cleaned was a task that I remained incapable of completing myself. It's a very strange sensation when someone else enters your mouth with an electric toothbrush and a heaviness of touch guaranteed to make your gums bleed. It shouldn't register as one of Britain's best loved spectator sports yet somehow we managed to make a very real case to start issuing tickets and charging for admission.

It's not easy to offer advice to someone cleaning your teeth when your mouth is full of their fingers and your toothbrush, particularly if you can't project your voice anyway. However when any new protagonist approached my mouth having been deputed with responsibility for cleaning my pearlies I always wanted to confirm that they proposed to turn the brush on once it was inside my mouth.

Failure to do this would result in projecting toothpaste at the very least across the person trying to clean my teeth, but on a couple of occasions covering patients in the beds on either side of me. Some nurses want your advice, others don't, considering my attempts to instruct them patronising. This either makes the person carrying out the exercise cross or prone to the wobbly chin giggles.

The evening performances varied in terms of the numbers in the audience but the record crowd was seven personnel.

Which made me mindful of a sort of anti-feminist joke 'How many nurses does it take to clean a patient's teeth? Answer, 7, that's one to carry out the exercise, 1 to write the notes, 1 to supervise, 1 to write the health and safety report, 1 to clean up afterwards, 1 to initiate the training exercise, 1 to review performance against government targets and 1 to share the experience'.

Of course if you're counting you will realise that makes eight, another reason the NHS finances are in such a mess.

It was all very well having the attention but it became even harder when one particular nurse, Sarah, explained that she had recently installed a computer at home and was worried about fluctuations in electricity supply. She had invested in a surge protector.

For some reason to my simple mind this sounded like a character from a film combining the best and worst of 'Allo 'Allo and Inspector Clouseau. 'It is I, Serge!' 'Surge who?', 'Serge Protecteur, you Fuhl'. To be pronounced in an absurdly French accent, of course. It wasn't that funny but it took a full half an hour to stop giggling, and three weeks before we could talk about anything else.

I had been trying to improve my French by listening to language refresher courses on CD ROM. In addition I had been trying to pick up Italian and Spanish phrases by talking to members of staff. My perception of the Philippine language was so hazy however that I did not dare attempt any one of their dialects or many tongues. For some reason the Spanish staff latched on to me as someone who could help them improve their English. They wanted to know who had the most quintessentially English voice. Naturally I turned to Terry Thomas whose over the top impression of an Englishman came to mind, transcending his Mersey origins.

I wasted many useful hours with a gaggle of Spanish staff around me learning to say 'You're an absolute shower' either in Catalan or a new tongue called Madridoise.

The results were not at all successful but the mirth was reward in itself.

'Be jubilant my feet' is part of the chorus of the anthem John Brown's Body. I heard this verse over and over in my mind hoping that by repeating it I might stimulate some signs of life in the lower part of my limbs.

It seemed of little use while staggering along a corridor with two physios in tow as I went for a promenade comprising a limited number of paces. Walking was such a tough thing to re-learn. There was so much to co-ordinate, the roll of the foot, pivot of the ankle, elevation of the knee, reflex in the calf, stride through the thigh and rake of the spine to maintain balance. It was extraordinarily tiring and relentlessly painful because neither leg matched the ability or pattern of the other and the strain inevitably got taken up by the back, where the muscles were starting to awaken from their enforced hibernation. This was all very well, and perhaps appropriate if walking along the seafront at Brighton where the challenge was entirely horizontal. To regain really meaningful mobility I needed to be able to get up and down stairs. So poor were the reflexes in my right leg that I couldn't even raise my right foot onto a shag pile carpet let alone a full height step.

Without grip in my hands holding on to a banister was difficult so the ever patient physio team would clench my forearms and talk gently into my ears like horse whisperers.

There was a tiny flicker of life down the inside of the left leg; one or two messages were clearly getting through to some of my toes. It was just possible to get this foot on to the step and with sufficient support on either side, stand while concentrating on motivating my left thigh muscle to take responsibility and elevate me upwards. My right side should have been ashamed of the paucity of its contribution but no matter what level of caution, bullying or encouragement was offered my dexter and sinister remained disenchanted with the thought of reconciliation.

The expression 'hard yards' would have aptly described the level of effort involved to summon a relatively paltry return but they were more like hard inches in terms of the physical achievement. There was some cardiovascular involvement, climbing the stairs always gets the heart racing but most of the time the obsession was just in getting muscles to remember what to do and how to do it. There was no easy way.

By repetition marginal improvement was achieved each session, the bar would raise it self in anticipation of achieving slightly more the next day. If you're fit and able-bodied it is impossible to picture a direct comparison.

All I could do was compare how I felt at the end of each of these sessions with how I remembered feeling after going on a five mile run, in my previous life.

I was starting to feel my age just as much in terms of my life span as in terms of the time I had spent in this hospital. Some of the senior sisters had become more than just caring, helpful people. A union had grown between certain key members of the team and Suzi and me. Not only were we part of the furniture, we were becoming the mascots!

We don't get older in equal units of time, each year marking exactly 365 days of progress. We get older in dollops! I was 28 for an awfully long period of time before I finally accepted that I had just turned 40, this of course at the age of 47 1/2. If this was my 50th year would I ever recognise it? Would I collect my £200 as I went straight past Go on my way to the Old Kent Road?

I knew I was much older than I had been before the illness struck. I would have to accept that Saga would now be writing to me regularly about Stannah stair lifts, coach trips to Eastbourne and a retirement home in the Algarve.

Life was never going to be the same again. But I was now in an altogether different world. Who was this new person whose washed out old body I had taken over like a soft crab seeking shelter in someone else's shell?

Questions bounced around in the head...Do I know you? Do I really know who or what you are? And how exactly did we get introduced?

Answers began to form but never became complete, it seemed too narcissistic an exercise... Too much self indulgence, too complicated and besides... here comes Nursey.

After ten years out of nursing, Liz had returned to her vocation. Deeming that her two daughters were now sufficiently independent to allow her to go back to work she set about her duties with a viagral approach (you know, always ready for action and firm in all the right places).

She was knowledgeable and skilled, caring and aware.

Within moments of arriving on duty you could taste a sea change in the attitude of the staff around her and the sense of being supervised.

Her warmth and humour were infectious and her preparedness to give Suzi lifts home in her own car at the end of the shift provided hard evidence of the philanthropy of her nature. She also managed to engage my brain in a way which none of the other nurses did.

She talked to me as though I was well again, dismissing the things that I still could not do for myself as mere triflings. A real cup half full person she reminded me of how I thought I used to be in my previous life. More realistically she probably just made me feel better about the art of being.

Instead of just thinking about the weekly unit of measurement forward and backward, certain dates were starting to loom as targets.

Firstly there was the prospect of my father's 90th birthday in the middle of July and secondly there was the concept of moving out of the hospital environment and into rehabilitation. With a lot of encouragement from the occupational therapy team and several practice runs I learnt how to get in and out of a motorcar from the wheelchair. At the beginning I found it impossible to swivel into the car without someone pushing me, could not adjust or fasten my seat belt, and had to plan my bodily functions well in advance to make sure that I was not going to be indisposed on any journey, far less this special one on the 10th July.

My father had fallen over and broken his hip some two years prior and never really recovered full mobility. On his special day we both arrived at the sweet little hotel near Bath on a scorching sunny afternoon determined to see who could strike the most immobile pose. Both of us required Zimmer frames and could barely stand for any length of time. I had never before witnessed my father writing a speech out in advance, he had always been consummate in his ability to stand up and talk to an audience with wit and panache. This time though he was anxious to thank all those who had not only helped him reach his ripe old year but who had also gone out of their way to assist me.

In Washington DC hanging in their National Art Gallery are seven grand old oil paintings depicting the ages of the development of man.

Each is equally spellbinding in the detail and imagination played out before you. They are set on a river, you journey down a stream which broadens and gathers pace in tandem with the expansion in size of the vessels that carry you until you reach a certain point where the journey starts to slow. I vividly recalled trying to explain to my children why I did not like their most recent choice of white noise music; as soon as I started the sentence I knew that I needed to slip my words into reverse gear.

Yet it was too late, the words kept tumbling out and I could not divert their course. At the point where I heard myself say 'personally I prefer something with a bit more melody' I knew that I had become my father. That would have been portrait number five.

It was particularly poignant for me therefore to witness my father stumbling over his words as he tried to read and repeatedly lost his place in the notes that he had so painstakingly prepared in advance. It was just so unlike him. Perhaps it was simply testimony to the decline in his powers as his years had gone on to such a grand old age. In the event he reverted to type abruptly discarding his notes with a peremptory 'Oh bugger this' before peeling off a cracking Joan Rivers story which brought the house down.

Two of my father's oldest friends from his time in Malta when he was on active duty had made the journey over from Suffolk. Agnes was still as immaculately presented as ever while Idwal her husband looked resplendent in his Prince of Wales suit. Time had caught up with his hearing and sadly he was almost completely stone deaf.

As the party wore on so the groupings fragmented and I found myself in the garden amidst baking hot sunshine resting in the shade underneath a parasol. Agnes and Idwal came to sit at the table nearby watching some young children playing croquet. The heat was starting to affect everybody and pretty soon they both closed their eyes. Without warning Agnes fell off her garden chair, hitting the grass with an inelegant thud.

Within moments every able-bodied young man was in attendance to winch her back into her seat, settle her down again and proffer a reviving cup of tea. For my part, my mind flew straight over to Agnes while the rest of me looked on, marooned in the GBS departure lounge.

In a Brian Rix farce this would have been deemed quite funny, but the most humorous part lay in the fact that Idwal managed to sleep right the way through this event and to this day remains blissfully unaware of his wife's travails.

I was very proud of my father that day for how he managed to get through it and his enduring choice of friends and companions.

I confess that I was also quite proud of myself for managing to be there and not disgracing the family in the process. They were all there, the cousins, the aunts and uncles, the godparents, the guardians, neighbours old and new, wives, sons, daughters, photographers and even a black Labrador.

Boy, was I tired afterwards and for the first and only time greatly relieved to get back to my hospital bed.

The splendour of the day seemed to clear the last remaining obstacle to the next stage of my repatriation. We had done our research thoroughly and discovered that there was no better place for recovering from neurological illness than a rehabilitation centre in Wimbledon. It is a curious fact that for all our investment into the private healthcare world, that unless your surgery choice is elective, the National Health Service is by far and away the best and, in some cases the only, recourse open to you. The next few weeks were all concerned with preparing for the big move.

The long goodbyes became very long indeed and the balance between rehabilitation and physiotherapy and a vaguely social world shifted towards the latter. One of the leading sisters who had taken especially good care of us throughout my stay was called "Scary Sarah". She was a tall, slim and elegant woman blessed with the most extraordinary manner at the bedside. When dealing with critical cases she was able to project tremendous empathy through her voice and body language. To my astonishment she started to cry when someone else told her that I would be leaving in a couple of weeks.

Apparently I had been a model patient and the ward in which I had been placed seldom had an inmate staying with them for so long, who had maintained an upbeat outlook no matter what the adversity.

So my acting skills had not deserted me after all!

I had assumed that they would wish to bring out the flags and bunting to celebrate my departure from the ward with loud shrieks of delight plus an Oompah band and a certificate from the head of the hospital saying 'Thank goodness you've gone'.

Not a bit of it! Almost every single nurse who had looked after me in the intensive care unit made a point of coming to visit me before I left.

I lost count of the number of staff ranging from doctors to the most humble part-time care worker who took the time and trouble to seek me out and wish me well. Ranging from Jason Gardner's mum, who works as an auxiliary, when not cheering on the 'Bath Bullet' to 60 metre dash victories for Great Britain all over the world; to the student nurse who lent me a book on metaphysics to pass the time more quickly. Time passing faster than the speed of sound had never occurred to me but page 132 soon put me right.

If you ever despair of human nature, of mankind's selfishness or the moral bankruptcy of lives that you observe, then I commend a slice of hospital life to restore the pleasure of absorbing values and beliefs that we should really never take for granted.

It was impossible for me to say goodbye to everybody but I did my best.

It is hard to describe the sort of bonds that you form with the people who are caring for you. The exchange seemed so one-sided. They kept on investing time and effort and work into me; while I felt so unable to do anything other than take from them. I was told this was not the case.

If it is your job to take care of people, then you get your reward and your return on your emotional investment through the improvement that you witness, together with the more subliminal messages of encouragement that your contact time with each other creates.

After Kirsten had been promoted to bigger and better things within the stroke patient world, Pam had become my physio mentor. She was the person who taught me how to climb the stairs. Very Scottish of voice, she was persistent and perceptive in equal measure. It was she who ensured that no matter how much physiotherapy we repeated each day it never really felt repetitive.

Thanks to Kirsten's training she knew what was required to make the treatment varied and interesting, always getting me to do more than I thought I could.

Pam went on holiday just before I left so we never had a chance to say goodbye properly. Yet the first document I should be presented with on arriving at the next rehab centre was a postcard from

Pam on holiday in the Alps wishing me good fortune. She was thanking me for being her patient.

Priceless!

As the months had worn on and we were heading towards seven months in the RUH so the reliance on food from outside the hospital had gathered pace. A menu that rotates every three weeks come winter, spring or summer can hold no more hidden delights after so much studious consumption.

Suzi had conjured up all sorts of meals at different times of day to provide the variety and the freshness so cravenly lacking from the standard fare. A Thai green curry here, a seared salmon with pesto breadcrumbs there, salads, fresh fruit to keep away the scurvy, all surrounded by looks of grave suspicion from fellow visitors and patients. I adored every mouthful.

One particular friend brought in delicious risotto in a thermos flask from time to time and my youngest son Charlie introduced me to the delights of the cheapest Indian takeaway in town. Known as Desh, the colouring of their speciality dishes had clearly been inspired by Britain's traffic light system; Red light for a mild dish, Yellow for medium and Green for go straight to the loo. To be fair to the hospital staff, they objected very little to our rampant rejection of their best culinary endeavours.

On the penultimate night of my stay in hospital Charlie delivered a Desh special and Sundance, Suzi and I savoured the delights of our Last Supper, with the lovely Amy, one of the indefatigable care assistants, playing wine waiter. Amy was one of those plucky souls with an impish face, a very pretty smile and an unquenchable thirst for hard work. We had managed to smuggle a nice bottle of Rioja in for the evening and thanks to Amy's loquacious skills she had blagged a bottle opener.

It was a very poignant evening, the end of an era.

Mentally it was something I was desperate for: to move onto a new challenge, to the next level of expectation and demand. Physically it was a big ask!

My body wasn't really ready for independence yet, but I had to try.

In my subconscious I knew that my time was up.

My treatment in this hospital had run its course and in spite of everyone's best endeavours I needed a different level of physical nourishment to get me better. There was just the small matter of leaving a huge piece of my heart there behind me.

Somewhere hidden in our deep subconscious we all have ambitions to leave something memorable behind. After we have departed this world a living epitaph would do nicely. Ideally it should enter mainstream awareness in society: perhaps a building, a work of art, scientific breakthrough or precedent in law which defines moral judgments for centuries to come.

Such thoughts of self-aggrandisement are usually the preserve of madmen and politicians. Admittedly the scale of ambition was much reduced on my part.

All I wanted was to select something suitable to thank all the staff for putting up with me for so long, that wasn't a bouquet of inappropriate flowers or large box of vulgar chocolates.

The solution eventually came to me after much consultation with the staff themselves. I confess there was no mighty drum roll, cutting of ribbons, or local dignitary to break a bottle of champagne open across a newly launched commode.

With a minimum of fuss three new office chairs, for their main reception desk, were delivered to enable every member of the team to sit comfortably for at least part of their day. They arrived quite deliberately after I had left.

Spike Milligan always wanted the expression 'I told you I was unwell' written across his tombstone. A friend suggested that I should have the legend 'Goldilocks and the three chairs' emblazoned on mine.

Why such morbid thoughts amidst all these valedictions? Perhaps it was anxiety. Possibly it was a fear of new levels of the unknown. More likely it was the sense of impending loss that brought home the realisation that after seven months in the same hospital surrounded by very unwell people, most of whom I would never see again, a reminder had been served.

It was a clear message that the dividing line that allows us to hold onto our mortality is so precious that life should never be about what objects we leave behind. Getting all those possessions through the eye of the needle to take with you is impossible.

In the end we shall all be judged by how we touched the lives of other people. It will be about their feelings and the emotions that stirred in them.

Perhaps the last thing that we do learn about ourselves is our effect but that doesn't mean we should not do something with that effect once we realise what it is.

Somewhere lurking deep inside us all there is a Good Samaritan waiting to get out!

CHAPTER SIX
SUMMERTIME AND THE LIVING IS QUEASY

The raid took place at dawn, two burly ambulance men laid me out on a stretcher, hurtled me into the back of an ambulance and whisked me in a straight line for London. The sun came up over Reading, heralding a brilliant summer's day as we arrowed toward the leafy glade that is Wimbledon. Quite unused to walking any distance before, I was welcomed with the instruction that this was a rehab centre and I should get myself off the ambulance and into the registration area by myself. It was precisely the next level up of physical demand that I needed.

The Wolfson Centre is a classic example of the sort of building we are now desperate to tear down. Presumably there is an architect somewhere who is immensely proud of his design of this building, who could drone on about the way the natural stone look and concrete had weathered together. To my layman's eye it was pug ugly. But it served its purpose well, wide corridors all very clean, polished seamless floors, perfect to push a walking frame along with all main facilities on one level and lift access to different floors.

I was placed in a room with five other men, it felt as though I was attending a United Nations conference. The fellow delegates were Mr Kwek Bong Hoo, Mr David Ndoo, Mr Salvatore Pucillini, Mr Bola Adebayo and Mr Jeremy Spector. At least there is one English bloke here that I can talk to, I thought.

Little did I realise that he was to become the 'fiddler on the roof'.

I tried very hard to walk wherever I could, pushing a Zimmer frame in front of me, remembering to keep my legs flexed, rather than to be stiff from the hip downwards, a 'cycling without a bicycle' technique I had begun developing weeks before.

In my haste to get around I was sacrificing stability.

On the first Saturday there I caught the edge of my walking frame on the mat by the front door. It had been placed there for health and safety reasons.

Well it wasn't safe and I didn't feel very healthy as I got my foot caught on the edge of the mat and fell to the floor with a mighty thump. Because I still had no powers of control over my arms, I was unable to break the fall. The back of my head cracked onto the concrete floor and my lights went out. Not only had the fall shaken me but it had sent my nervous system into overdrive.

I couldn't feel my legs. There was a shooting pain in my ankle. I couldn't feel my back, yet my ribs were smarting.

I was frightened.

The very same devil who had danced the jig of delight on my tongue all those months ago when I first collapsed made a most unwelcome return. The head is the king of the body and I was incredibly grateful that my thoughts and conscience had hitherto escaped the battering that had stormed the rest of me. Now there were flashing lights, thunder claps, florid helixes and sirens laying waste to my composure. Perhaps it was Machiavelli choreographing the tango, so invasively performed by the Antichrist as my trepidation turned to panic. I was seeing stars all right but they were not from a friendly galaxy.

I had become used to a lack of communication with my body but this assault on my nervous system was more personal than that, it was affecting my brain and I could not and did not want to cope with the maelstroms.

My constant companion Suzi was at my side, in a trice. But then she started crying and all the bottled up hysteria of the previous months came spewing out. We wept uncontrollably. She tried to prop my head up on her arm. She was wearing a little Prada number, a stone coloured cardigan.

The cardigan started to turn a wondrous shade of claret, as the back of my head bled copiously. The crash team arrived and determined that I should get straight to the casualty department of the local hospital.

Now I don't recommend downtown Tooting at the best of times, but 10:30 on a Saturday night in accident and emergencies is not my idea of Nirvana.

I was the only outpatient there not in handcuffs!

Everybody else was attached to a policeman, high on drugs, roaring drunk or plain abusive.

There is a certain twisted logic in the suggestion that our current police stations should be abandoned and transferred to a building adjacent to every accident and emergency department in all of our national hospitals. This may well be the most pragmatic option but what a desperate, sad indictment of the society which we now live in. I was not a criminal and objected strongly to being lumped together with a posse of felons. Do I want to live in a world where suffering an unfortunate injury places me into an arena so intimidating in its hostility and so alien in its dyspeptic culture? No, I certainly do not! So you will understand why I was so keen to leave this battle zone with or without conclusive evidence that my brain was still intact.

Please just get me out of here ...

After making unnecessary jokes about how easy it was to get blood onto a stone (cardigan) my head was glued together again and we drove back to the Wolfson Centre, in the dead of night. The sense of relief was palpable.

I was kept under strict surveillance for the next 48 hours. This made it difficult to sleep. I was woken on the hour every hour to check my blood pressure and pulse. If that had been the only interruption perhaps I wouldn't have minded.

I had been moved to a different room to avoid interrupting the United Nations conference delegates at rest. They had also moved Jeremy into the room with me; our beds were divided by a lime green and blue curtain. I was vaguely aware of a small amount of activity in the next bed which became more and more urgent, noisy and intrusive. I was absolutely desperate to sleep but 'the fiddler' had started his concert and was determined to put on a fine performance. As the level of thrashing escalated and the vinegar strokes approached I found myself willing my roommate on to his musical climax.

At last the end was reached, the sighs subsided, the bed stopped creaking and peace broke out. Surely now I would get back to sleep after such a tiring day.

To my horror he started again. I could not believe it. All sorts of envy about the strength of his libido and jealousy of the fact that his hands worked and mine didn't, were banished. Now I was just plain cross and roared at him to behave. I might as well have been talking to someone from Venus, or on the roof, he just carried on regardless.

The following day I was told that Jeremy was suffering from memory loss, and could not recall whether his mother was alive or not. He could still play the piano beautifully, and often did at the old Joanna left in the canteen, (he had once been the musical director of a concert hall) but missed a note around the one in ten mark. His wife was very concerned for him, understandably, but did not feel she could cope with him back at home. She asked what it was like to be in his company and to share a room with him. No, I didn't think about telling her the truth, I proffered some vague blandishments and wished her good luck with her deliberations. I felt so sorry for both of them, not knowing which to pity the most.

After the first two days of assessment to establish precisely what I could not do, the physio team set out an escalating programme of exercise each day which was principally focused on my trunk and legs.

For instance, standing with my feet together unsupported was beyond me, so when asked to do this with my eyes closed I fell over. Turning around once in a circle was out of reach, walking backwards impossible, getting up from the bed without help a task too far. Flexibility in my core was almost non-existent and touching my toes out of the question.

Responsibility for my arms was abdicated to the occupational therapy team and the head of the department Sarah introduced me for the very first time to quite the most wondrous device I have yet to see in any institution, let alone a hospital. I was about to put the Robin into Heath Robinson. The 'OB Help Arm', to give it the official title, comprised a series of pulleys, strings and levers suspended from a metal frame which was manoeuvred in over my head. My hands and elbows were then clipped into leather pouches to support my arms. Counterbalanced by weights behind me I felt for the first time since my relapse as though I could move my arms by myself.

You may well have lost the use of part of your body through perhaps a broken leg or dislocated wrist. It is painful, inconvenient and very frustrating. I am not looking for sympathy but trying to help you understand the sense of total inadequacy.

When you lose the arm and hand function completely on both sides of your body you need to rethink your approach to everything because 95% of the things that you used to do for yourself are now beyond you. That is why this was such an extraordinary moment for me. It marked the very beginning of becoming independent again.

Almost weightless it was possible, although not easy, to raise a hand toward my mouth. The scriptwriters for Thunderbirds would have been very proud of my impression of Virgil. To all intents and purposes I was a puppet on several strings. A broad grin took over my face because I was just so excited. When the muscles are wasted and exercise fatigues them rapidly, the new motto has to be little and often. Back and forth to the Help Arm I would go four or five times every day.

Progress was not quick but then I had stopped expecting any rapid advance. My expectations were built around the weekly measure. By sticking to this rule I knew that life at last was starting to return to my upper limbs.

The OT department had their very own workshop replete with workbenches, and panoply of tools. By now I was moving around the hospital with a Zimmer, in short staccato bursts, shuffling along with a grating sound which enabled anyone to hear me coming from miles away. Thus by the time I got to the workshop all equipment could be laid out ready and waiting. There would be half an hour of arm exercise at the workstation, then half an hour to recover, before returning to the workshop. Simple repetitions like sanding a block of wood with an abrasive edge over a painters' easel, across my body, then up and down, from side to side ten times, change hands and repeat. Or grasping different shaped objects buried in a bowl of lentils, lifting them out then returning, to wake the senses of Rip Van Winkle's nerve endings. All enabled by suspending my arms from the OB and defying gravity with several tightropes but no safety net.

There was an adjacent open terrace cast out of concrete with no redeeming architectural features at all. Favoured by those patients who craved cigarettes it was paradise for the smokers. My walking was still not strong but I had enough strength to shuffle the Zimmer frame back to my wheelchair which was lying out in the sun.

That terrace was not attractive to most but it was as pretty as Audrey Hepburn in a cocktail dress to me. You see, it faced southwest and attracted sunshine throughout the day.

I became expert at sunbathing in a wheelchair. This may not seem like the most interesting hobby to indulge in but the front of me benefited greatly from a daily dose of vitamin D while the back of me remained a familiar pasty white colour. If you can remember one of the early scenes from the iconic movie The Graduate you will have a good impression of where my mind transported me while splayed out across the wheelchair. By closing my eyes I had taken Dustin Hoffman's languid place as Benjamin lying on a clear plastic Li-Lo in his parent's swimming pool. Refusing to entertain any of the exhortations to get off his back and off to work he preferred to fritter his time away in the California sunshine; listening to Art Garfunkel harmonising with Paul Simon on their way to Scarborough Fair. This seemed like a pretty good place to be, and certainly beat the reality of life without use of your hands.

I was trying to spend as much time in the open air as I possibly could. The regime here was not harsh but it was exacting, goal oriented, and quite clear that I was to be there for three months and no more. The culture was very different from the previous hospital.

Everything was designed to encourage you to take as much responsibility for your recovery as soon as you were able, independence was prized.

The daily curriculum was exact: to be washed and dressed at 7, at a table in the dining-room for communal breakfast by 8, off to the first physio session by 8:30, lunch at 12:30 and dinner at 6. Everyday there was a fixed gym session at 1:30 which included such delights as the exercise bike, the parallel bars, stretches and contortions on a bench and a warm up routine which I will always remember.

Our group of about 10 would sit in a circle on harsh metal chairs, each of us suffering from various ailments in our own special way.

We were all hopeless at each of the activities, yet the competitive spirit surfaced to such an extent that you could see little personal battles taking place between the stroke victim in her 70s and the alcohol induced stroke victim in his 40s practising how to stand upright from a sitting position.

Each was desperate to do one more than their immediate neighbour.

Somehow this made everyone look as if they were Jonny Wilkinson waiting to take a penalty kick for the England Rugby Team. Just like him we put our hands together in front of us, set our feet wide apart and pointed our bottoms towards Plymouth.

The supervisors provided music and work out routines customised for each of us. We still managed to fall off the running machines and burst colostomy bags in the fall or start punching the walls as an epileptic fit set in. It certainly wasn't graceful or truly aerobic like a trip to Champneys ought to be but it was vital for all of us to try, to take part and to 'think well' again.

Anthony was a bricklayer by trade and Chelsea fan by obsession. He boasted a shaven head giving him the air of the archetypal unsavoury and aggressive football fan. He had suffered a series of seizures over the past 18 months which had caused a stroke down his left side. Pressure had built up on his brain forcing the surgeons to operate on his scalp, opening it up over the top of his head from left ear to right as though a zip belonged there. How misleading first impressions can sometimes be, for Anthony was a really gentle man.

He went out of his way to help anybody else around him and was for ever opening doors for female patients, proffering chairs in the dining room and offering to run errands for the less mobile. In the exercise sessions he took it upon himself to ensure that a chair was ready for me to sit down on, not just any old chair, mark you, but the only one in the room with arms. I was easily the worst in the group at standing up unsupported when I first joined the sessions. Thankfully I became more proficient over time. Graduating to the chair without arms was a singular and most gratifying achievement.

These sessions became the fulcrum of the day. I tried to increase the strength and pace of the repetitions to create a cumulative effect. My first attempt to sit on the exercise bike involved three people lifting me on and one staying with me to ensure that I didn't fall off again. Initially I was unable to stay on the bike for more than five minutes and ride for half a kilometre, frequently having to stop along the way. After nearly three months I could last 25 minutes without a break and cycle 10 km. This is not meant to impress, it's not a great achievement in itself but when you multiply the progress in this activity with an equal level of improvement in all other disciplines it gives some idea of the journey you have to take your body on.

Mind you, it took me a whole day to recover. On many days I just overdid it and paid the price either by losing my balance through exhaustion and falling over which is painful or becoming too tired to carry on. Learning to pace oneself is part of the discipline.

If you don't do enough you barely improve and if you try too hard it is all too easy to harm yourself.

For Anthony it was about earning a living. What he needed to be able to do was to hold a brick in his left hand so he could apply the cement with his right. Is that too much to ask from life? His brother brought bricks in for him to practise on and some days he laid a few, other days were more difficult as the hopelessness of his plight hit him and the tears of frustration overflowed.

I miss Anthony.

Rather like the two curious black diesel engines from the Thomas the Tank Engine children's book series two Duncan's appeared in the hospital at the same time. It was easy to see the difference in personalities, one was dazed and confused, while the other was confusing and crazed. It was important to identify them separately so the new soubriquets of Duncan Disorderly and Duncan Doughnuts arrived to join up with them like goods vans. Both had suffered strokes down their left sides so their speech was relatively unimpaired and they could feed themselves with one hand.

Disorderly had an impossible triple-barrelled surname. His memory loss was profound, although in his business life he could remember that he had created a wine museum near Borough Market. He was desperate to, and fully believed that he was going to return to develop more of these museums around the world. He was particularly keen to open one in Beijing. He had psoriasis in all of his fingernails and was useless at doing his clothes or shoelaces up. His new saturnine demeanour was the antithesis of the urbane and cultured man that he had obviously once been.

Doughnuts was funny. A broad Glaswegian, with a once brilliant financial mind he had made and wasted a fortune. The demon drink had taken a stranglehold on his outlook, preventing him from making any sensible business decisions from lunchtime onwards. His humour had remained razor-sharp although his memory was distinctly selective. He kept cracking jokes and spotting the opportunity for a gag.

A typical example occurred when I once exclaimed that I would love to see the Wallace and Gromit film 'The return of the werewolf (rabbit)' which prompted the following riposte:

'We know a story about that don't we, children?... I used to be a Werewolf, but I'm all right naooooooow...'

His blood sugar levels were shocking to everybody except him, so staff were deputed to prevent him from sneaking a biscuit or obtaining sugar to put in his tea. His previous addiction to alcohol had mutated into a fresh addiction to sweetness. The former had nearly killed him. The latter would almost certainly finish the job off.

Doughnuts latched on to me at meal times. It was important to ensure that I sat on his right-hand side as we only had his right-hand between us to assist with the feeding process. The dining room was a communal area for all patients to eat in and spartan in the extreme. The days of being spoon fed at, or in, one's bedside at the first hospital were long gone. Everything here was designed to make you try to help yourself and I was as willing a participant as the OB Help Arm could make me become.

Thus I could get to the table and if the chair wasn't too low sit down to wait for someone to push me in and stick a napkin around my neck.

I still needed to be fed as I couldn't take the OB into the dining room to get my arms to lift but the return of sensation in my shoulders enabled me to nudge plates and cups with the side of my arms.

Over the weeks the team, and Doughnuts, enabled me to graduate from total reliance upon them to a curious halfway house. The vanguard of this journey began with a piece of toast. The index finger and thumb of my left hand started to show small signs of movement; even though my biceps hadn't caught up. I was able to grasp the edge of my first granary slice and by rocking my body backwards drop my left elbow below the height of the table. This lever system popped my left hand upwards with the toast pincered in my tenuous grip, enabling me to drop my head over the toast and munch my first piece of marmalade splattered Hovis. Frank Cooper's finest it was not but it tasted like 'Sheer Ambrosia' to me. Admittedly a lot had gone on to the floor and much on to my T-shirt, but there was no mistaking; I had managed to feed myself independently for the first time.

Slicing food with a knife or spearing it with a fork was still way beyond my compass.

However by wrapping handle enlarging foam grips around a spoon I was able to grip (or rather rest cutlery in my hands) and with crude lunges induced by my shoulders shovel food around the plate before utilising my newly perfected lever system.

It was important to try and raise my arm and hand up to 45 degrees and dive down over the food swiftly, any higher angle or dawdling on my part and the food was on the floor. It was barbaric, vulgar and grotesque to observe but a vital step in reparation. Polite society would have to wait patiently for my return. If manners are supposed to maketh man then this man was making up his manners as best he could.

For a while people seemed quite reluctant to come and sit next to me. I wondered why, but not for too long, because the feeding environment was becoming an arena in which to experiment with miniscule changes in my dexterity. Almost any food was up for grabs to find novel ways of getting it somewhere near my mouth.

I drew a line at the custard though, it was radioactive! Bright orange by day they had to lock it away at dusk, it used to glow in the dark!

The food was clearly prepared off site by a centralised cook/chill system to ensure consistency of standard at the lowest point imaginable and a complete lack of culinary intrigue every time. Once in a while the chill system broke down and the two girls retained to do the finishing off of the cooking process had to improvise by doing some of the actual cooking themselves. The food that they put together was just great, flavoursome, fresh and zestful; in fact it was the exact opposite of the food they spent the rest of their working week dishing out. Why do we spend our lives in this country centralising the control of brand standards ranging from cooking to shopping? Is it to keep the accumulation of wealth in the hands of the few? Or to remove the risk that once in a while something might go wrong?

Well the net result of this particular centralisation was that we seemed to be removing the risk that something might go right!

Usually the highlight for the cooking team was writing out the menu on a white board with a green felt tip pen. It was certainly a highlight for me because the girls wrote down the components of the meal as they came into their head rather than the usual sequential order.

Thus if you were trying to decide what you wanted to eat for lunch you could elect to have peppered chicken casserole with chocolate sauce or lemon tart with garden peas. It was hard to decide whether the greater challenge lay in selecting the food than consuming it, although as my patent pending lever system became more sophisticated the odds changed.

There was a reverse curfew after 6 PM which allowed patients to leave the building provided they were back in reasonable time to get to bed. The summer was turning distinctly Indian so most evenings offered a wonderful blend of heat slowly evaporating from the warmth of the day, cotton wool clouds meandering by at a lazy pace, long shadows and shafts of golden sunlight in the park on the edge of Wimbledon Common named after a Sicilian nobleman called Cannizzaro.

This hidden gem of well balanced tree selection contrasted starkly with the scrubby nature of the rest of Wimbledon's common Common. It was tucked in behind an hotel which was in the process of being sold, and refurbished at the same time, which gave it a real identity crisis. Less than five minutes by car from the rehabilitation centre it was possible to find a park bench easily from the many dotted around the perimeter of this deciduous enclave. It was at this hotel that I met up with Mike Harvey, the old college chum who had suffered a cocktail of illnesses to which the addition of Guillain-Barre had been the last straw. What united us now was not the devastation that our respective illnesses had wrought on our, and our partners, lives; but the first straw, because neither of us could drink without one.

We looked like spiders from Mars as we blundered our way out of wheelchairs onto our sticks and frames and crabbed our way past normal people to collapse into chairs which had the word comfy writ large on them.

Listening to his partner Nicola's fulsome tales of sedulous support for Mike through thin and thin made me feel like a total poltroon, by comparison with the brave and relentless workload that she and Suzi had put in to rescue their men. It took her words to articulate all that should have been said between Suzi and me, but which had remained unspoken because we were too busy doing the doing bits. Mike was remarkably upbeat but claimed to have retired from his previously helter-skelter working life, ironically running the catering for the hospitals of Hertfordshire.

We were looking at each other warily, as though we were mirrors reflecting our souls and inner psyche. Typical men unable or unwilling to put anything but a superficial sticking plaster on our emotional wounds. It was familiar but disquieting, too old muckers having a catch up. So many things were left unsaid. There was too much ire in our hearts to enable the initial flummery of conversation to turn into real, deep, meaningful sense.

Two broken souls were simply having a tangent before returning to their parallel shattered lives.

The thickness and variety of the mature trees planted around the perimeter of this park created the very clear impression that we were deep in the heart of the countryside. Admittedly the planes flying over to Heathrow in the distance were a bit of a giveaway, but the wind direction often took the noise away from the park so it was still possible to suspend belief.

There were acers and elms, mighty oaks, limes and magnificent spreading horse chestnut trees, copper beech, london plane and weeping willows and not a single leylandaii in sight. Cannizzaro House had a terrace which was the perfect spot from which to view what felt like a very private but capacious garden. Dogs set free from their leads bounded and sniffed their haphazard route defying their owners every exhortation and yet somehow invariably mimicking the manners and appearances of their guardians. Kites swivelled and perched above the tree line offering dramatic swathes of colour and movement against vivid blue skies.

There was a sense of bliss that could enshroud you each day, often only fleeting, yet it was there to be savoured as you absorbed the panorama that offered its embrace. Sometimes the park could be full of people without ever feeling crowded or that your style was being cramped. Suzi was as ever by my side or pushing me or just being there for me, enabling me to sample life albeit from a pick and mix format. She transmitted her strength of spirit by deed and word, still with her own life on hold and no chance of earning any overtime. I was not an easy charge.

Yet style was something I possessed in abundance. I looked resplendent sitting in my wheelchair with a picnic basket rested upon my withered knees. I knew what a dash I was cutting!

When you are in hospital people expect to see wheelchairs and so have no need to hide their surprise. When you are out in open territory removed from the safety of the hospital environment you present most people with a different challenge, except children. Able-bodied people are embarrassed by people in wheelchairs. They don't know how to respond, whether to avoid eye contact, smile engagingly or somehow convey the 'I'm sorry for you and know how you must be suffering' look in their facial expression. It takes practice and few of the British public have done much training.

As a wheelchairee I decided to take the initiative and avoid people's stares, unless I was laughing. In which case I would look directly at anybody walking past me because I knew how relieved they would be feeling to see someone who didn't make them feel self-conscious.

Children however are quite different, they speak what they see! If they spot you being pushed along the grass they will invite anyone within hearing distance, including you, to tell them why that crippled man is in a wheelchair. 'Why don't his legs work?' The answer of course is to ignore the question completely and attempt immediately to distract the child by engaging them in the hopelessly random subject, that has just come in to your head, about something that neither of you have ever shown any previous interest in before.

Getting out of the building and into the world of the well is such a vital component in the recovery process. It is all too easy to accept one's new-found status as a victim of circumstance and to give in to it. You can become very self-conscious, frightened to confront the normality of an outside environment and intimidated by your own perception of your inadequacies. In short, being disabled makes you antisocial.

I wasn't having any of this whether my appearance shocked others or not.

Going to the park was relatively easy because you didn't have to sit too close to strangers and was quite a gentle way to begin the readjusting process.

Restaurants were an altogether different prospect, and I set off for my first Sunday lunch in Wimbledon high Street with a childhood friend called Nigel, whom I had known since we were seven, who had returned from Australia for this very meal. Nigel's three children had been born in Sydney and he was wrestling with the pipe dream of returning them to England. It was great to see him. The humour was still intact, the self mocking deprecation unharmed by 25 years of Aussie triumphalism, and he emanated happiness. But three months of fighting the M25 later his mind was made up and he returned to the allure of the barbecue. The dilemma of whether to change out of his work shorts into his evening shorts once home, in which to char-grill a shark or sear a kangaroo, had proved insufficient a barrier. The beauty of the Wolfson Centre just fell short of the view of the Opera House from his back garden.

Getting the Zimmer frame between tables, finding a chair of the right height, which wouldn't slip on the floor as I tried to sit down and push back into it, holding the menu, unwrapping a napkin, lifting a glass or twisting the pepper mill... these were all new enormous challenges in terms of detail, yet seemed like mere trifles when set against the task of pretending to be a normal person. You so desperately want to be the same as everyone else there but you are not, you are a bit of a freak show.

The adults may pretend not to be staring, skilled at averting their prying eyes just at the moment when you realise you're being stared at and look up to return their gaze, but not children. Kids just look at you as only children can and talk about you as though you are not there.

They know who the fakes are and they had me well spotted a mile off.

CHAPTER SEVEN
BRAIN JUICE

The glamorous Vera, a good friend of many years' standing, interrupted her international jet-setting lifestyle to go on the Internet on my behalf. Her detective work was sound and she quickly tracked down the Possum 7210.

This mighty beast perfected over many years of trial and error was built to handle books and periodicals for people unable to use their hands. It turned pages electrically!

Angled like the top of a lectern it was attached to a stand which had an electronic touch pad on top. Once seated in front of this page turner I was able to activate the machine by pressing my chin against the pad. It could turn pages back and forwards but sometimes shuffled a couple of pages through at the same time, but that was a minor nuisance. At last I could follow a story and pretty much go at my own pace; Cry Freedom indeed. I kept at it and made minor improvements until after weeks of practice I managed to get my left thumb propped over the pad and begin manual operation. My right thumb was still studying for his masters' degree in shyness and showed no signs of jealousy that his traditional place in the pecking order of duty had been usurped.

The question was where to site the thing? It wasn't exactly small and discreet. There were two principal lounge spaces in which all the patients were deposited between their appointments. The main room was a cavernous space completely dominated by a six-foot wide television screen in one corner. Well worn armchairs, none of which matched any other, were pressed hard against the four walls, leaving plenty of space for the patients in wheelchairs to be carted in and out.

It was a desperate space and one in which I really did feel most uncomfortable.

The television was always on so loud that you couldn't have a conversation with anybody else there and the battle for stewardship of the remote control waged constantly. I had never watched daytime TV before and have no desire to repeat the experience. To witness the passion which some of the inmates showed for a programme about twelve men, 11 of whom were gay, trying to fool a quite pretty young American girl into choosing them over the rest of her courtesan suitors seemed quite iniquitous. We were acting out our own soap opera; there seemed no need for extra rations.

Next door was an altogether smaller room, known affectionately as Fish Lounge because it had a fish tank in it. Not that there were ever any signs of fish moving about in the tank, just the usual parade of bubbling water, pebbles and miniature ruined castles. There was a compact television screen, which was turned on occasionally, plenty of books and reading material together with just the right space to park my machinery.

By placing the page turner in a corner of Fish Lounge I staked out my territory.

On reflection it was quite a hostile act.

Not quite on the grand scale of invading Poland, or sending all those Russian tanks into Czechoslovakia one sunny Wednesday afternoon. I was effectively saying 'this is my study, visitors are welcome by appointment only' and as I had found in the previous hospital one's status elevates, by and large, according to the length of time one has been in an establishment.

So Doughnuts and I composed a poem to mark the occasion of the page turner installation. Quite dreadful in its pacing and use of rhyming couplets, we gave up after welding the following tribute to a drop of sherry in the afternoon.

It's called Xerex, which is pronounced Hereth.

XEREX

Perfect palindrome or sweet briar,

Milk, cream, oloross or amontillado,

Scoop from the schooner, tongues on fire,

Shipped in casks to Bristol promenado,

De La Frontera, Brunel bound with Harveys,

Loved by old ladies, the navy and the armies,

Bang out of fashion, save for Withnail and I, who matter not a jot,

Is that Romulus or Remus craning to sip a hearty tot?

I know, you're right, it doesn't get better in print. But at least it took our minds off the reason we were there in the first place.

My very first meal in the dining room had proved the sadness of our demise conclusively. I was invited to sit at a table with a gentleman who did a brilliant impersonation of Martini from the Cuckoo's Nest film. Rotund and short, he had a hairy chest which came up over his shoulders forming a complete link with the hair behind his head and showing no signs of a break at the front of his neck. He was wearing a bib under this chin not to keep the growth of hair in check but to prevent the food falling out of his mouth from ruining his shirt.

I tried engaging him in conversation several times and after the fourth attempt caused him to burst into tears. This wasn't because

I was being rude, or unkind. It wasn't because I was asking tough questions about the meaning of life or whether England would have been a nicer place to live without the effects of the enclosure act. The poor man couldn't talk!

What a bastard.

I must have seemed as though I was on some kind of cruelty kick.

I just did not realise. He was so frustrated by his inability to talk that all he had left to express his emotion was to cry.

Outside the dining area watercolour paintings produced by the inmates adorned one wall. You've guessed it. The artist with all the gold stars on his work was the very same man. Known as Kahn he made me feel very humble. Life seemed to disturb him in unexpected ways and I came to realise, in time, that it wasn't just me who made him cry. Everything did.

When you're the new boy and just finding your way around you need to make friends quickly. Replenishing lost childhood dreams with Kahn through Friends Reunited did not seem a likely outcome in the future. So I latched onto Royston.

A real South London geezer, Roy was on his fourth marriage and had fathered 15 sons. Not one single girl amongst them.

He didn't like being teased about eating more white meat, or adjusting the way in which things hung in his boxer shorts and he wasn't taking any jokes about King Herod either.

Roy had been in floods. To him a bit of damp spelt work. A misplaced downpour, while tragic for some, mixed with a few missing roof tiles was a certain recipe for soggy carpets, insurance claims and lots of mess to clear up. This was Roy's forte, to him the disaster at Boscastle was a glorious opportunity. A bit of water seepage from the first floor into the living room was his wet loss adjusters dream.

I shared a room with Royston and we scratched along just fine. Royston was what was known as a 'character' but underneath the rough diamond exterior there was a kind and compassionate fellow who would make friends with anyone. He was the usual sad story of a stroke victim paralysed down his left side. Five years of trying to get his left arm to work independently and remove the splint from his left foot, had made little impact. Yet he played golf to a level with one arm every weekend down on the south coast, wrapped everything that needed two hands to do it up in Velcro so he could tie shoelaces, trousers and bags up with his right hand and compensated for his tilt to the left by walking with a stick. Learning new ways to put clothes on by putting himself into them, rather than get half dressed; he was a triumph of simple mind over matter.

Nothing seemed to get him down because in his world of positive mental attitude everything was just "laaaaaavly".

Royston also liked a bit of a fry up and set up the breakfast club for 'gentlemen only' every Thursday morning. Occasionally some ladies were invited provided they agreed to be gentlemen through the meal. Picture, if you will, a group of eight men with two useful arms between them bumping their Zimmer frames, prosthetic legs and sticks into each other, in a galley kitchen.

Each jockeyed for position to get as far away from the actual cooking as possible. More Daddies sauce and ketchup ended up on the floor than ever did on the breakfast table. Royston's house speciality was eggs over easy, over easy, over easy! Because once he started flipping the eggs he found it very difficult to stop. My principal contribution to the first breakfast was to get out of the kitchen and to sit down.

My school report at this stage would surely have been too condemning to show my parents.

Somehow my confidence grew and I graduated to the washing up section of the duty roster. Because I couldn't pick dishes up I developed a sliding technique to prod the dishes along the work surface and nudge them into the washing up bowl, stirring the murky fluids around with a shoulder induced twirl of my fairy brush.

Perhaps it was the water that helped me regain this misplaced confidence. It had certainly helped me discover freedom of movement in the pool in the RUH.

The hydrotherapy in this hospital was much smaller than the one in Bath and there were no invasions of coffee mornings to get in the way. The physio team here took turns to look after me, although Anna, the head girl in charge of my case, proved a constant touchstone through my time there. I don't know why I decided to lie on my back, and set off on a reverse butterfly motion, probably instinct. I doubt that I will be representing my country in this new discipline but the level of freedom derived from arching the arms to the side, then straightening up over my head and down again through the water had a wonderfully liberating effect and if you were in a wistful mood a certain 'Don Quixote's Windmills' look to it.

All my time in the water felt as though it was stolen because it suspended belief and reality. As soon as I got back out of the water I found it became impossible to replicate anything like the amount of movement I had just enjoyed in the pool.

On one particular morning Fiona, a fiercely fit and desperately hearty physio, took my hydrotherapy session. She was very determined and cajoled me into a whole raft of new movements.

At one point, when she was trying to make me jump backwards in a somersault and to bring my feet up above the level of the water, she implored me to attain greater levels of exertion with the following memorable lines 'Go on, get it up there, make me happy, go on, get it right up there now, you can do it... That's it, yes, yes, yes!'

I asked her if she had ever thought of becoming a script writer for a porno movie. The joke died as soon as I cracked it. I don't think she ever realised what she had said.

Her focus was on my wellbeing. To get me able-bodied again was a target that united us and I was hugely indebted to the practised skills, methods and can-do culture that she and her colleagues relentlessly supplied.

Other friends were desperate to help and in an effort to give Suzi some respite from attending to me every day a number of buddies volunteered to look after me. Amongst her best pals Lesley and Michael, Pete and Di, Julia and Colin, Fi and David supported her as much as they so kindly nurtured me. On one particularly delightful Saturday an old girlfriend of mine from college days who lived nearby, called T, collected me from the Wolfson, placing wheelchair and Zimmer frame into the boot of her car and whisked me away to the delights of Richmond Park. Originally the principal hunting ground for royalty it is now arguably London's most attractive thoroughfare. There are cars everywhere. By this stage in my recovery I could manage short distances pushing a Zimmer frame out in front of me but found it particularly difficult wherever the terrain was uneven. So we set off in the wheelchair dodging the deer, cyclists, joggers and golfers looking for miss-hit balls.

There were black clouds in all directions save for the spot of blue sky directly over our heads and we enjoyed a totally unfettered time as this shaft of sunlight led our march across the park and back again without getting wet. We rested a while on a small pedestrian bridge and played pooh sticks.

Or rather she threw the sticks into the water and told me which one was mine!

When set against the problems that my fellow patients had to endure, such opportunities to recapture one's zest for life made me feel like a very rich man indeed.

No one could say that I was alone in my solitary confinement with so many offers of help, ranging from the support of my family to work colleagues, from new friends to old allies with whom bonds were forged decades before. In this the hottest of furnaces in which to test affections, were extra layers of gratitude and thanks tempered and shaped. The strength of ties previously untroubled had well and truly been stretched. For this I was so much more fortunate than many, but there were other cases around me that were so harrowing I felt blessed to be who I was, in spite of my infirmity.

So fast was I running out of Brownie points to award those who had helped, as Suzi had qualified for 99% of the quota, that I decided to switch to Brownie point 'futures' to loosen up the market.

Unlike the previous hospital the centre admitted patients who had a much wider set of reasons for their infirmity. Winston, a powerful and athletic Caribbean man, had been waiting for a routine operation. The administration of the anaesthetic had gone wrong and he had been left substantially paralysed in parts of his body and unable to stop shaking everywhere else. He constantly tried to talk yet was unable to articulate anything that closely resembled words. Nor could he adjust the volume of his mutterings.

You become hardened to such intrusions when you sink back into your private world but Winston's case was a desperate one. His wife and daughters came every day to administer food and help, displaying such fortitude and strength of character, in the face of the horrifying adversity that Winston presented them with.

One of the patients looked like Charles Manson. With long grey hair, sallow skin and a tattoo on every knuckle and every limb he was an intimidating sight. Jack was confined to a wheelchair because he had been attacked in a pub by a madman with an axe and a screwdriver. He had punctured his lung and cut through a nerve in his spine. The bloke who did it was arrested the same day following this attack and two further assaults which had become murders. High on narcotics, he had embarked on a drug fuelled rampage either emasculating or terminating other people's lives indiscriminately. He left Jack obstreperous and difficult to deal with. He needed help, yet did not want it, and his dyspeptic ways intimidated the staff. No one ever volunteered to look after him; he was trouble.

By comparison with his partner Linda though, he was a pussycat. She was clearly an addict and impossible to have a normal conversation with. Hyper, neurotic, erratic, prone to tears and downright weird, she plainly still loved her man but could not give him the comfort and tenderness that he craved, partly because his appearance hid his need for affection so well but mainly because she could not cope with looking after herself let alone anyone else.

I studied Jack's hands and noticed that the left-hand had the word 'love' spelt out on the four fingers. On his right hand was the word hat. I made the mistake of asking him what happened to the missing e. 'Got bored' was his first reply. Before long, though, a smile slowly started to break out across his face and very quietly he whispered to me, 'besides, I am very partial to a bit of e.'

Many years previously I had studied a day release course at the Dundee College of further education. For some bizarre reason I thought it would help my post-college studies to become a member of the Institute of Personnel Management.

In my first year there we studied sociology, psychology and statistics. On Monday afternoons a disparate band of students would unite to broaden their minds. The subject matter would give 'paint staying wet' a run for its money in the dullness derby, but we fella's kept going because of some very soft cashmere. Dressed in an always ivory white jumper, Ali's pneumatic breasts enjoyed cult status as they held the male students' gaze for the entire duration of the lectures, save the odd interruption from the person in charge.

Occasionally she would speak and we were all torn because the lilt of her Kirkcaldy tongue, the urchin haircut and the retrousee nose were all beguiling attractions which added an extra lush to her lusciousness.

Each component was worthy of its own fan club, but the eyes could do nothing to stop man's appalling ability to compartmentalise women from taking control; and soon the breasts would take centre stage again. What a handicap.

I sat next to a charming boy called Martin Cleghorn who was attending the course because his father told him to, and who was in total awe of the cashmere queen. He worked in a cloth manufacturing business in Dundee and hoped one day to succeed his father by owning the family business.

However Martin had not covered himself in glory when first deputed to the personnel department of this factory because he had failed to follow set company procedures to validate job applications. Not only had Martin employed a 60-year-old triple axe murderer, who brought shame and dishonour to his father's company, by committing the crimes during company hours; but unwittingly Martin had employed his son who then went on to complete his own triple axe murders as well. Even worse, this was during working hours too.

If you're going to commit a triple axe murder you should at least have the decency to do it in your time off. Somehow the 'triple screwdriver' tag doesn't have the same ring to it. We kept in contact for many years and Martin always used to sign postcards to me with the witticism 'Yours as ever, Jute the Obscure'.

I really could not work out whether Jack would have been better off becoming the third murder victim of his axe and screwdriver brandishing assailant or eking out an existence confined for ever in a wheelchair; cast adrift in a permanently fetid orbit following his most hostile nemesis. It troubled me for days, almost becoming as troubled as Thomas Hardy's hero.

Then I came to realise that Jack would have continued to abuse his metabolism by consuming every substance that he could get his hands on; flagrantly challenging his body to process alien drugs and support his well-being as if he were leading a healthy lifestyle with a balanced diet. There would have been no turning back.

His 17-year-old son came to visit him dressed almost exactly in the style of Donovan, the eponymous 1960s folk singer, on the days when Linda was not present. I studied the interaction between them. The son had become the guardian to his own parent. How much and how quickly the boy must have had to grow up to fulfil the role that his father was no longer capable of. How much the father now relied upon the son, in a complete juxtaposition of his former stance. Perhaps as much as the Wolfson had come to rely upon the work of one man.

The whole of the centre ran on proficient lines because of the huge affection that its principal held for the centre. Dr A, most definitely a character created by Peter Sellers, (a combination of Dr Strangelove and an Indian Raj) was a lovely man much admired by all of his staff and adored by those patients able to recognise his extraordinary powers of humanity.

Apparently without social life or family to comfort him when away from work he never seemed to leave the building and had the uncanny knack of entering any part of the Wolfson unannounced at precisely the point when his presence was needed most.

He rarely spoke directly to you because he was a painfully shy man and preferred to speak to people by talking to an area high up on the wall over either one of your shoulders. Eye contact was therefore rare but was compensated for by a dry humour and an abundance of compassion.

At first glance you might suspect him of being an incidental figure floating along the stream of life in some misanthropic way, but this would be to miss the substance of the man. His encyclopaedic knowledge of all his patients, former staff, current charges and supernatural eyesight for any situation which might need his presence were extraordinary.

The way that the staff gravitated towards jobs within the centre demonstrated that our tribal instincts are not yet dead. The physio and occupational therapy teams were without exception of Caucasian extraction, well-educated and middle-class. Those that did the catering were from deepest African countries desperate to escape military coups and mass slaughter at election time. Irish and Philippino staff tended to do the hands-on care assistant work, making beds, washing patients and pushing you around in a wheelchair. None of them ever complained or went into a huddle to moan about one of their colleagues. They were all unfailingly cheerful and united in a seamless way to ensure that the very special needs of the patients remained the permanent focus.

The patients came from all walks of life and their case histories were fascinating to me.

Carol was in her early thirties blessed with two charming young children and an incredibly patient, and supportive husband from New Zealand.

She had suffered two aneurysms which paralysed her down the left side and forced her to retire to a wheelchair. Her features were so dominated by flowing tissian hair that you knew immediately that all her family stock was from Ireland. The paralysis through her left leg and arm came up into her face giving her mouth a lopsided smile. One of the main reasons for her debilitation was the effect that smoking had on her arteries.

The message did not get through to her conscience though and every opportunity she had to get a cigarette into her mouth she grasped with the one good hand left to her. You could tell that as a school child she had always been the naughty one hiding at the back of the class. There was a wonderful air of mischief about her which made you feel in conversation that you were both about to get up to naughty little tricks. The renegade atmosphere that she created was contagious, mixed perhaps with a hint of sedition from Huckleberry Finn and a dash of Catcher in the Rye?

She started to go on home visits at weekends to see how much adaptation of the facilities in her house had to be made by social services when she finally left the hospital. At home her husband sensibly did not allow her to smoke, causing them to argue fiercely. It was desperately sad to see all that love exist between them and yet witness two people lashing out at the person they cared about the most.

I realised how fortunate I had been to get this far through my recovery process without losing the emotional plot or allowing the overwhelming egregious nature of my decline to get the better of me for any meaningful length of time.

I could not have done this on my own. Thanks to the implacable nature of Suzi we kept our spirits up, kept being positive and always found things to celebrate and savour. I had a nice view to look at every time she appeared but she got the short straw, she had to look at me!

It wasn't easy; ebullience was not a crop that could be easily harvested in the field next door, the process was too enervating for that.

I looked back to one particular point when two friends, Stuart and Tony, had bowled down the motorway to visit me from Manchester, ushering in their raucous sense of humour and reducing me to mirth just at a time when the misery gremlins were drawing in.

Whilst admiring the top of my head they asked me how the physio was going. I started to bore them rather about the minutiae of my daily exercise regime when they interrupted me, 'We are not interested in the physio you're doing for your body, how is the physio going for your hair? Surely you can't go around with a hairstyle like that without needing someone to exercise it and make it do trunk curls?'

Don't worry, I will get them back one day, but their determination to force me to laugh at myself was an ideal tonic; almost as ideal as a special day in the country.

We were invited to a day out in the Oxfordshire countryside which involved a journey of almost 1 1/2 hours duration each way. This was by far and away the furthest we had travelled from the hospital and a real test of our organisation skills, my bladder and general stamina. As we arrived at the village cricket green we were welcomed by a lamb roast which had been cooking slowly since breakfast. It looked and smelled divine. To one side were dotted lime and oak trees laid out in a random fashion. It was a soporific scene, efficacious in the extreme.

For our delectation a grand spectacle was being performed utilising some white and some not so white items of clothing, wickets, bats and balls; together with 30 highly unfit family members, long lost uncles, nephews and nieces; plus the odd ringer, hired assassin and semi-professional.

Normally there would be 11 characters per side but this was a day for extraordinary substitution rules to enable everyone to take part no matter whether they were boy or girl, able or not. The cricket may have been a joy to watch, but it really didn't matter because there were so many other things to soak up, while the sun caused a shimmering heat to rise above the tree-line. This was a world I had not seen for the best part of a year; The British countryside in full bloom, in late summer and looking as capricious and becoming as I ever remembered.

Blossom on the trees, overflowing hedgerows and leather on willow, lazy butterflies and the clink of fine bone china tea cups; all these sights and sounds combined to remind the senses of the diversity of pleasure that nature gives us for free. Pleasures which we too often studiously avoid in our desperate dash to get to work on time, attend meetings, and make things happen as the adrenalin courses through our veins making us as high as junkies.

I was busy getting stoned on the panorama as I beheld a full colour 3-D world as if I had just been released from watching black and white television for months on end. Participation would have to wait. What a privilege it must be to walk unaided, to hop skip and jump, drive a car or butter your own scones. Deep down this day etched in my conscience; the certain knowledge that I had never once realised how lucky I had been for 50 years of my life to have enjoyed such consistent independence of movement and thought.

How I wanted it back.

The main event, however, was not the cricket match.

Whilst I had settled down into a deck chair two young children aged 6 3/4 and 5, commandeered my Zimmer frame and turned it into a leisure centre for the entire afternoon. They used it as a climbing frame, ran races with it and through it, creating their very own version of the Highland games in the process.

These two youngsters showed remarkable ingenuity as they fashioned hours of pleasure out of the frame. In a trice the young girl turned herself into a Dalek carrying the frame around her shoulders and issuing instructions to her younger brother. Do as you are told or I will be forced to 'exterminate' she commanded.

As soon as her back was turned the young boy picked up the frame, flipped it on its side with the wheels facing downwards and pushed it along like a wheelbarrow. The window into their world was wide open and unashamedly I stared right in, savouring every moment of their innocent delight.

As the heat started to evaporate from the day and the sunset began its slow descent Suzi and I set off back to the Wolfson Centre.

Not much was said on the journey, we both knew what a special day it had been and that another substantial rung in the ladder had been scaled. I wasn't miserable when we got back, just pensive, and very aware of how institutionalised I had become.

So unused to the wideness of the outside world, I had been shut off, incarcerated, hidden, forgotten and squashed by this year of years.

Hospital rooms were the norm, not expansive vistas or delicious panoramas. Disabled people were my peer group, not happy adults and children frolicking in the fields.

Life had been happening to me while I was busy trying to make plans. I wanted my life restored. This mugging had taken it away from me. I was not going to rest until I found it again.

If cricket seems to be taking centre stage too often at various stages in this tale I make no apologies. For this was the year in which the Ashes were regained.

This was the year when England finally managed to lay the various Australian ghosts which had haunted them since the 1980s in their attempts to prove themselves at the highest level of the sport.

It also happens to be one of the few sports which you can pick up and put down through an entire day as the ebb and flow of either sides fortunes juxtapose.

The pleasure may only have been vicarious but it was definitely visceral as Freddie Flintoff captured the hearts of many previously uninterested, sport avoiding people. The margins were very thin between success and failure, but that doubled the pleasure for a partisan Englishman such as me, because the Australians came so close to snatching victory from defeat. Sport was being played out at the highest level to be judged by the finest of margins.

Like most Englishman my pedigree is a bit mixed, with French Huguenot on one side, Irish and Scots on the other. Indeed, unlike many current day Muslims, I hadn't actually been born in the country. I was Maltese. George Bernard Shaw once described Malta as Europe's largest unfinished building site and he wasn't far wrong. If Malta had been a man it would have been Sid James in a string vest talking about work that needed to be done but never completing it.

Finishing things off was a characteristic of the people of Gozo, the better cared for, verdant and less blousy little sister of the two islands.

Yet Malta possesses one key thing: it has history, shed loads and boatloads of the stuff. Most of it based around the two key harbours on either side of the neck that supports the head of the island, its capital Valetta. Grand Harbour in particular is, as its name implies, the most magnificent amphitheatre in which to dock, repair and float your boat. Any ocean going liner of any meaningful size can only be put fully into context when moored in such a cavernous bay.

The honey colour of the sandstone, the turquoise of the water and the azure of the sky enable any ship in its opalescent white uniform to shine.

Like busy ants serving their master 'Dghajsas' (pronounced dicers), the indigenous small craft of the island, scurry around from one duty to the next in a complex series of weaving patterns. At the head of each of these boats an eye is painted to ward off the evil spirits of the sea and the rest of the craft are coated in shades of aquamarine, blue, yellow, green and red. Images of these boats have remained in my mind since childhood. We had left Malta on a long northbound journey up through Sicily onto the foot and shin of Italy before traversing across Europe and returning to England.

My parents had decided to return home when I was aged three. Little did I know what a poor exchange this was in terms of weather. The real loss though was of my deep-rooted love of these native vessels.

In a child's mind these boats had a life of their own, a life on the ocean wave. In which the main part of their job description was concerned with keeping a watchful eye over the sardines, mackerel and occasional dolphin that inhabit the Mediterranean Sea. I had always believed it was also their duty to watch over me. We all have our God, I suppose. These inanimate craft, no matter how rudimentary, provided my first lesson about man's need to worship something.

Religion wove its way through my recovery, beginning on the wards during my time in the hospital in Bath, in many varied but fleeting ways. A pious father from a Benedictine monastery who had remained detached from the toils of the real world since the end of the Second World War proved the most uncharitable companion to have about the place.

This quixotic man had the opportunity to make an impression on all the other unfortunate souls nearby in his ward. He chose to carry on as though he was adhering to a vow of silence in his monastery and spread no Christian kindness by deed or word. I accept that his stroke had debilitated him and caused hardship.

Yet he was patently more mobile, able to talk and give to his newly found brothers in arms than anybody else in the adjacent vicinity. To him we did not appear to exist; perhaps he was offering silent prayer on our behalf, I doubt it. I saw more evidence of Good Samaritan work from hundreds of people around that hospital than I ever saw from Father Donald.

Each Sunday night there was a service in the chapel and volunteers went into every ward in the hospital drumming up support for the service. I joined them on some evenings and on others just sent my spirit instead.

Sally was a near neighbour of my father's and visited me regularly, partly because of the personal connection but also because it was her job as a volunteer.

She helped the hospital chaplain by making pastoral visits to all wards in the hospital, aiding those souls who were lost, supporting those who were nearly found, and facilitating for the few who were knocking on heaven's door.

Making peace with your god whoever he may be is not really fair when you are in desperate need.

You should cut your deal when the stakes are more evenly balanced. Yet life rarely works like that, because you only know when the vacuum exists in your life at points of high drama or great loss. Not too many have access to God's fax number for rapid expressions of repentance.

Elaine was a very pretty girl from Frome who camped in our ward next to her husband's bed for six nights on the trot. He had been experiencing some muscular problems and had fallen down the stairs in their new home. The truly concerned relatives and friends were allowed to ignore the rules of visiting hours and stay on-site pretty much throughout the day. Night time, though, was not a normal period to see visitors around so it was particularly concerning that she should need to keep up a 24-hour vigil. The marriage had not been going well lately and the tension between this handsome pair was sad to behold. An athletic and powerful man in his early thirties who had just started his own business when his health gave way, Mark was troubled. He was overwhelmed by her desire to make things right between them when deep down he knew that her guilt was the motivating factor.

They started to pray together, offering what tearful oblations they could. At nightfall as the lights were softened in the ward they pulled the curtains around Mark's bed and Elaine laid out an air mattress on the floor. They held hands and spoke at length to their Lord. Moaning in the gloaming!

Sometimes religion comes along and smacks you in the face. Sometimes evangelists take it upon themselves to impose their religious beliefs upon you. Sometimes God seems to have deserted you. Sometimes your belief in one creed is so overwhelming that you will commit heinous crimes in misguided support. For me I was finding it difficult to believe in an afterlife; unsure if I did whether to return as an insect, the county of Gloucestershire, a piece of wood, or Keith Richards' right hand. Because I was unconvinced, not knowing whether I had already died and come back for a second go as a poor impression of myself.

I didn't feel at peace with my God. We were on speaking terms but not the same wavelength. I still hadn't found the answer to the semi-secular question which had dominated my thoughts for months on end. It wasn't a long question it wasn't particularly complicated, it just needed a straight answer...........Why?

After putting her life on hold for so long, Suzi had at last been persuaded by her girlfriends to take a few days off with them... such temerity, how dare she go away and be normal, it's heresy, I say, a grand treasonable offence!

They had flown off to the French Alps. A swell time was had by all and after relaxing for the first time in months she returned to England and decided to take a shower before coming back to the hospital. She reached up for the soap and her left arm flopped to her side. She tried again and the arm collapsed in the same fashion. Being the practical person that she is, there was a moment or two for composure before calmly moving the left arm around her head again this time with easy movement. When she got to my bedside she was upset and tearful, there was clearly something wrong and the nurses and I persuaded her to seek help. She was rushed away.

I went to see her staying overnight in the hospital awaiting tests. It was a scene of reversal, Suzi making light of things, but now the patient being tended by me in a wheelchair being pushed by George, sequestered into her own first floor room. There was no immediate conclusion; after various theories were proposed several possible outcomes were left open. It was weeks before the conclusion was reached that she might have had a small stroke or trans-aschemic attack, the doctors weren't sure... the pressure was telling on them and us!

It wasn't just the facts of the matter, it was the injustice... how had my demise triggered such a stress related response and that pernicious little question to pop up again...why?, why?, why?

It just was not fair. She had worked so hard to prevent me giving up and maintained such a fantastic serenity and evenness of mood throughout, that I was far more upset for her than I had ever felt for myself. Here we were in hospital with every conceivable testing aid available and still we could not be sure what had happened or what it might lead too. What lesson was God teaching us now?

Religion didn't enter the curriculum at the Wolfson, we had the Archers every Thursday instead.

For an hour we had poems, recitals, stories and jokes read to us by a character actor who has for almost 30 years played the same role of Nigel in the institution that is Radio Four's indomitable incarnation, the Archers. Gamely he would play out his thespian role but we were a challenging audience. We never clapped or laughed in the right places. We nodded off during the punch lines and were incapable of summoning an encore. He was playing sweet music inside my head though and for that I will always be grateful. In itself his words were not particularly poignant but his tune was redolent of a bygone era when I had no fear of my own mortality and reminded me exactly of the moment when my first puppy dog Holly, aged six weeks, chose to come and live life as a Sheppard, selecting herself from a litter on a farm in that village. Yes, that's right, the village in which the Archers is set. He provided the catalyst to help my mind fly up and away from the rehab centre and back into a comfort zone of pleasures past. It wasn't a sententious interlude that he provided but a chance to re-connect with ones beliefs and, dare I say it for some of us, uncover our faiths.

Yes faith was there alright, written indelibly in the beliefs of the vexed relatives, the volunteer helpers, the patients with an ounce of optimism and in the handbooks of the senior staff.

When faith slipped out of my grasp, from time to time, I found it incredibly difficult to cope with the levels of sadness. Sadness that sat like a foggy shroud as it surrounded me amongst my peers and supervisors. How I longed for the time when I could take my dog for a walk along a country lane, and throw sticks while trying to catch the wind and shoot the breeze all at the same time.

My body still wasn't ready to leave this hospital but, just as I had found towards the end of my time at the last hospital, I was starting to feel my spirits become terribly restless and in need of change. Amongst the more recent patients admitted to the centre were three men and two women who had experienced operations to their heads. This had left them with sizeable chunks of their skulls now missing. To the experienced hospital worker this is not surprising but I could not hide the fact that I found this harrowing in the extreme. The college report which claimed that my attitude to one particular subject had 'given rise to grave disquiet' now made sense. For the feeling that I experienced as my stomach knotted each time I looked directly at these new fellow inmates was undoubtedly one of disquiet that was ever so grave.

Peter was a very cheerful soul, diminutive in stature, big of heart and kindness personified. Part of his scalp had been peeled back to remove the offending growth leaving a lunar landscape on top of his head. He mocked himself by saying that 'You don't need a clear night sky to see the moon anymore.' During the gym sessions we took turns to go up and down the stairs. Peter was much better than me at mounting the staircase, except that he needed to wear a cyclist's crash helmet lest he slipped.

When taking those turns to scale the 21 steps I needed someone with me at every point, both up and down, and a seat at the top to rest and hold onto so I could turn round. I could not imagine a life with such limits permanently in place.

But for Peter his head was far from fully recovered and would take years and several operations before it looked anything like normal again. That was the prognosis from the outside. Inside his brain Peter was struggling desperately to recover his speech pattern. He kept the words coming out all right but they rushed out far too quickly and with woeful enunciation. The poor man became incredibly frustrated because it was so difficult for him to make himself understood. His impression of the opening lines of "Four Weddings and a Funeral" was as foul mouthed as Hugh Grant's early salvo of invective but with too few 'fcuks' and too many 'buggers' to warrant his replacement. Indeed if one chose to be super critical it sounded more like 'muck, muck and guggers', which of course must provide great comfort to Hugh. Such a doughty challenge to his top spot was being consistently repelled at the Wolfsons very own casting studio.

The side of Peter's brain which was still functioning perfectly could not adjust to the loss in translation from one side of his head to the other.

He found concentrating extremely difficult. Television was all right but reading was dreadfully hard work so I used to read to him from my electric page turning library. We raced our way through The Kite Runner.

We delighted in the joys of The Shadow of the Wind and became rather disillusioned part way through the Da Vinci Code. At the three-quarter way mark, this book moves from a reasonably paced and vivid plot with 'blockbuster movie' written through every page like a stick of rock into a stodgy mess with a poor finish and a storyline which unravels like a second hand ball of wool.

Our exclusive book club changed, however, as a number of other patients wheeled their chairs in alongside us or flopped down into an easy seat on which to rest their weary false limbs. We had an audience! Now our book club grew and the two lounges divided in culture. Doughnuts and Disorderly were regular recruits as too was Keith, a once prolific journalist, who in his fondness for beer had unsettled his constitution so that he had lost his right leg while his left side succumbed to the stroke paralysis so prevalent of fellow inmates.

The larger sitting area remained full of people wrestling for control of the remote buttons to switch TV channels. Meanwhile in our smaller study the once erudite and learned atmosphere was fragmenting as the number of attendees rose and the banter escalated. Generally I would start out reading to others only to be interrupted so often that to get beyond one chapter was a rarity.

I switched from novels to poetry. Thankfully no renditions of Xerex but a bit of John Donne, Roger McGough or Linton Qwezi Johnson would prove a nice appetiser before a burst of Lord Byron, William Blake or Pam Ayers for main course. One common denominator for all poetry though lies not in humour. Great poets often write after bursts of severe depression or exposure to pusillanimous sadness. Our fulminating group could be rendered silent if a particularly poignant line struck the right cordant note.

There is poetry in pity and we were a pitiful and piteous audience. More power to the pity perhaps!

It may have been in pity that the charitable trust funding on which so many of today's hospitals are based first started, but there was no doubting its continuing effect. The Wolfson centre was founded on just such charitable finance, which would ring fence the property for another 50 years. The building was dwarfed by the remains of the vast Atkinson Morley hospital which once boasted majestic, now archaic, Victorian architecture. The estate had been reviewed by the trust which was currently responsible for the hospital's future.

After much debate, investigation and various studies the obvious conclusion was reached that the land on which the hospital buildings currently stood was worth much more if knocked down and converted into housing. Similar decisions have been made all over the country; Selling England by the pound indeed. The mistaken cost of which we will rue for generations to come as the national hospital land bank disappears and their property based reserves perish permanently.

Our bedroom block was surrounded by workmen feverishly laying down the infrastructure to allow what were once staff houses, operating theatres, canteens, wards and private rooms to be bashed about or torn down. Like an oasis in the middle of the desert our curious rehabilitation centre will remain unbowed for generations to come. An isolated island in a sea of des-res sprawl. To be surrounded by off plan salesmen, show homes, Bosch cookers and duvet diving conservatives.

Although still incarcerated at the Wolfson I was becoming much better at travelling short distances by car. I became used to getting out and about every day while developing ways to relearn once simple tasks like pulling the seatbelt across my chest. This involved a combination of putting the back of both my hands together on either side of the belt and using my chin to apply the grip when compressed against my shoulder. Adapt and adopt was the latest motto.

There were pockets of improvement in my bodily functions such as mobility in my shoulders and relative strength in my triceps. I overcompensated hugely with the bits of me that worked to make up for the recalcitrant parts that still didn't. Thankfully there was a compounding effect so that a marginal amount of additional strength was being generated every time I stood up from a wheelchair or sat back down into it.

My shoulders still dominated all upper body expressions of movement but there were definitely signs of uprising and potential overthrow by coup from my lower biceps and a couple of fingers working in dysfunctional defiance . I believed absolutely that I was improving, unlike a larger than life character who knew his future would only get worse. Bola was a big black man from Nigeria with an even bigger laugh. He had problems with advanced arthritis in his hips, a mild stroke and an operation which had gone wrong. He wasn't a well man.

In order to get around he needed a stick and someone in attendance in case he had one of his dizzy spells.

Even though life was not going to get better for him he managed to invest happiness into every waking moment of his day and spread his warmth and candour evenly across all those he met. Sure he was lazy, sure he was a little fruity with the ladies, sure he was terribly forgetful yet the cumulative effect of the weeks that I knew him will live on.

I haven't seen him since I was at the clinic, yet his cackle still sits there just behind my shoulder, booming out in raucous fashion like Long John Silver's parrot as a constant reminder that laughter is an essential component of the healing process.

We discovered that we shared an equal passion for a television series which had first hit Channel 4 several years previously. Thanks to a good friend a boxed set of the first series of the Sopranos together with a DVD player had been given to me and we were able to watch episode after episode back-to-back.

If you don't know the programme then I commend it to you. The story is based on a New York Mafia mob headed up by one Tony Soprano who cries wolf with his psychoanalyst about the difficulties that he is experiencing in his career which he euphemistically entitles 'construction'.

By night he goes out shooting people and by day he sits on a psychiatrist's couch ruminating on the trials and tribulations that his 13-year-old son is experiencing during the growing up process. 'I think he might be hanging out with the wrong kind of guys' from a fretful father contrasts marvellously with the epic line uttered when about to push a rival hoodlum over the edge of a suspension bridge into the murky rapids hundreds of feet below 'Consider yourself lucky, punk, I am in a good mood, I ain't going to shoot you on the way down!'

I knew all about the way down, as just to break the monotony I would fall over from time to time. This would always coincide with the point in the day when I had either overexerted myself in physiotherapy, or tried to move myself or something in haste. What I wanted to learn about now was not the way down. It was the way home. There was nothing cruel intended in my heart but it was evident. I knew I had been "hanging out with the wrong kind of guys".

I was becoming distinctly unimpressed with hard floor surfaces as I kept landing on them. It was that vision of carpets which overwhelmed me as one unsuspecting Tuesday we just quietly slipped away from the Wolfson, out of hospitals, out of rehabilitation and out of institutionalisation for what I hoped would be for ever.

Fat chance!

"Talent beyond words" - Andrew Eliel, past Editor 'Egon Ronay Guides'

*** *** ***

"Sad and giggly in equal double measure" - Helen Dorridge, 'Sydney Herald'

*** *** ***

"What an eye opener... just received a demand from the Inland Revenue which confirmed, if I ever needed reminding after reading these memoirs, that 'What the hell, health, true friends and family are the most important things in life as we should know it" - Tony Greco, 'Warrington Guardian'

CHAPTER EIGHT
AUTUMN LEAVE

I love the sound of Autumn

Translucent noise in September.

Linament smells for sportsmen's thighs.

Turf that springs under foot and hoof.

Dewy and ripe, not sodden.

Breath condensed.

The first morning snuffle in the nose

Leaves that crackle, bursting with auburn burnish

Oxford indigo night sky

Splashed with ploughs and bears so bright

Glow-worms, unwitting, perform Swan Lake

Tortoise shells anoint faded lavenders

Bucolic hazes fade and imperatives appear

In the crushed concertina that is Libra and Scorpio

Things to be done, resolution, fitness beckons.

The year is starting - work can flow now -

Before crumpets and wood smoke enmesh our aspirations

In the charcoal, fug and brine of winter...

After ten months of hospital life I was absolutely ready to come home. I was desperate to swap polished lino floors for a bit of tufted Brinton. The boot camp regime was finally over but I was still far from ready to be repatriated fully into society. There was a whole new status quo and a completely fresh set of partners, co-workers, supporters and carers to adjust to.

As Suzi and I departed the Wolfson with a significant volume of devices, props and equipment, the principal object which I hoped to render unnecessary at the earliest opportunity was the wheelchair.

Twenty years previously I had been to Marrakesh to collect a debt with a good friend of mine. After a couple of dark coffees at the King's very own hotel, where the staff walk along sweeping the gravel paths behind you to maintain an utterly pristine environment, we turned out into the madness and mayhem of the Souk. The noise and smell hit us immediately as the rest of the senses were assaulted by visions of snake charmers, sultana pyramids, aromatic spices, mountains of delicious dates weeping their oil, all covered with flies. Stalls made out of tomato or orange crates with rough hewn sheets across each trader to protect them from the harsh glare of the sun. It was a cauldron of excitement in this most vestigial, primitive market square which vibrated with colour, life and intrigue.

A broad shouldered man 'walked' diagonally across the square on his knuckles, he had lost both his legs from the thigh downwards and had strapped two old tractor tyres with pieces of string around the remaining stumps to enable him to manoeuvre across the dusty surface like a giant gorilla. His knuckles were gnarled and heavily calloused as they took the brunt of his weight. No one batted an eyelid.

They were quite used to the vision of this quadruped moving with lithe power in his very own urban jungle. To him a wheelchair would have been a Rolls-Royce option. The sort of option he couldn't even imagine because his country was too poor to consider the provision of a wheelchair as a basic standard of living.

How dare we take such things for granted in our civilised culture?

In a fit of absurd naïveté, I wanted to be able to discard mine and dispatch it to a Third World country where it would be treasured as a rare commodity.

Setting my target firmly to become independent as soon as possible I wanted to walk whenever I could. It was crucial to graduate beyond the boundaries of stamina and balance which had, hitherto, prevented me from travelling very far on foot, before having to resort to the wheelchair to complete any journey of substance.

Each day I went to the park by the river Thames striving to increase the range and pace of my walking. Still using a Zimmer frame my walking was hesitant over uneven surfaces on which falling leaves, twigs and yapping dogs became new opponents. I kept pushing my limits until one grey day when I completed a circuit of 1 kilometre around the park too quickly; my knees gave out 10 yards from my imaginary finishing line. The frame fell away from me and I sank onto my knees in exhaustion and self pity. Suzi quickly found volunteers.

With help from two strangers I was hauled up again and shuffled my way to the car. My frustration could be no more than short-lived as there was just too much assistance to call upon. If you knew where to ask and the right sort of questions to pose, an extraordinarily deep level of support was on offer. The local council were not going to let me back into society without help for the mind, body, sole and soul. The checklist went on and on. From such basic necessities as a bath board, to a frame to sit around the loo with arm supports in the right place to enable me to get myself up from what was still a very low height.

Can you imagine sitting on the loo and then not being able to get up from it without someone to help you? Yes, I was still that needy and utterly dependent on the clemency and compassion of friends and family to facilitate so much for me.

Additional banisters were mounted on the staircase, commodes delivered, finger splints supplied, crutches specially adapted with wide handles, adjustable height trolleys to enable me to eat a meal, placed close enough to my chin to get the food in without dropping too much on the floor. And so the list went on.

A phalanx of physiotherapists, occupational therapists, social workers, care workers and busybodies queued at my door to book time in my weekly schedule, thus starting the first tenuous steps of repatriation into the bigger world.

Kenneth the Portuguese carer, of African extraction, was assigned to visit me three times a day. For him I was a bit of a treat. He had never come across a patient coming back from illness before. He specialised in tending the terminals; those going the other way without hope of rediscovery or finding the person they used to be.

Kenneth is now my friend.

I grew to care about him as much as I grew to care about the fellow disenfranchisees left in life's ashtray or wastepaper basket by savage illness and blight, who were swept up and plonked into the 'system'.

The HQ for their repatriation into an alternative life was a community centre near Fulham Football Club close to the River Thames.

This was a day-care facility for people with a wide variety of disabilities which provided an essential crutch to the middle section of so many people's daily routine. Discarded by society because of their illness or infirmity, this building and its programmes helped put a little self-respect and purpose back into their shaky world.

The first wheel-bound patient in the building to introduce himself to me was Philippe who did up the top button of his shirt like a man of 75, drew multicoloured pictures with felt tip pens like a child of 5 and spoke to me in a covetous way as though we were both errant schoolboys of 15 who had just raided the tuck shop. He was in fact 45 and at the age of 25 had been in a motorcycle crash which had left him with severe memory loss and paralysed from the waist down. When asking my name he explained that he would probably have to ask me again in another 15 minutes because no matter how many times I repeated the answer he would not be able to remember it.This from someone who could speak Italian, Spainish, German and French underlined the tragedy and obscenity of his enforced sequestration.

He did however have one very interesting maxim which he applied when making any acquaintance. He would study the person that he was about talk to and then tell that person about the things which he had spotted and which he most admired about their demeanour and dress. This should have been a lovely way to guarantee that he could bring some happiness and warmth into the world of those people who looked after him.

Most of the time it worked well but one of the other faculties which Philippe had lost during the accident was how to gauge the difference between rude and polite. Thus 'good morning Margaret, I admire your cashmere cardigan, compassionate countenance' would start off well enough before taking a horrendous turn in the wrong direction by adding 'sultry smile, sweet smell and your lovely big bouncy tits!'

I liked Philippe.

The community bus would pick me up most mornings and zig-zag its way back to the Sunberry Community Centre where the waifs and strays, malcontents and unfortunates would have the quality of their lives marginally improved by a medley of activities. They would while away their days nourished by the care, love and attention of an army of philanthropically minded social workers.

The building was designed to induce gloom but despite its best attempts was not allowed to succeed because the ethos and spirit of the team that worked there would not allow it.

Here I would be deposited, waiting for the next bus on the relay to collect the hardy crew who wanted to conquer the equipment at their gymnasium south of the river. Conversation was always a bit hit and miss because you were never quite sure whether the person you were talking to could remember who you were and in some cases who they were!

Once on the bus a different culture wrapped itself around you. This was the sort of bus that as children we used to chuck 'V' signs at while the spaso's went past; now I was on the inside poking my tongue out and waiting for any sign of digital insurrection. My fellow passengers formed a patchwork of deprivations. There was William, ten years into his Parkinson's disease whose every move seemed so tortured. When he strode out he looked like the special adviser to the 'Ministry of Silly Walks', so over exaggerated had his walking pattern become to compensate for the debilitation of his illness. Sometimes his perpetual twisting and turning stopped as he went into the refrigerator. This could last 2 minutes or 2 hours, you couldn't hurry it or break it, you just had to wait. To me it looked rather frightening but to William it was just another inconvenience to tag onto the bottom of his long list.

When it was ready, and not before, his body would release him from this state of freezing and his heavily compromised participation in life could start again.

William liked cigarettes and sick jokes. The sicker the better; his favourite involved the tale of an old man admitted to a nursing home who is befriended by a lady called Doris who each afternoon makes him a cup of tea before placing her hand under his nightshirt, and holding his willy on the edge of his bed.

Doris is distraught when she realises that she has been usurped by another patient called Mabel. She confronts her former beau by asking him what Mabel has got that she hasn't. He replies that she makes me a cup of tea like you used to and she puts her hand under my nightshirt to hold my willy just like you used to... but now it is much more exciting because she's got Parkinsons!

Coming from anybody else this joke would be deemed to be in very bad taste, coming from William you had to laugh... for crying would hurt too damn much.

There was Dan the Dustman who couldn't read or write but compensated fully for his lack of these skills by talking the hind legs off as many donkeys as he could find. He craved attention and affection, wanted to put smiles onto people's faces, yet consistently missed the mark. It was his way of coping.

At 62 he had by his own account a highly desirable collection of toy cars and trains but insufficient boxes to put them in. My donation of empty Ferrero- Rocher clear plastic boxes for him, in which to display the toys, reduced him to tears. Dan did not live in a world overly blessed with kindness. Please don't ask who gave me the full boxes in the first place, they have their pride, and no, it wasn't that friend from Essex.

We all had our own methods to get by, some were constantly introspective, others absurdly loquacious. It was every man for himself in the 'how to survive disability' warzone.

No matter how much lifestyle coaching you offer anyone there is no one easy way to compensate for levels of debility that turn your world upside down.

There was young Keely who at the age of 20 had fallen off a roof and broken her back, to learn that she would never walk again and was paralysed from her stone encrusted tummy button down. You could tell that she was yielding to it though; the stomach for a fight was not there.

Oblivious to the effect her lack of endeavour in exercise was having on her body and constitution she would try to get by, pretending that nothing life changing had happened.

That was until she announced that she was pregnant.

This was a shock and awkward surprise to all who knew her. Who in all conscience would want to get a woman already in such a medically parlous state 'with child' and how in any God's name did they think she would be able to give a baby a future worth having. It beggared all belief.

Travelling independently I was often met at the Douglas Bader Centre by a number of other sorry tales; all tugged at the heart strings in equal measure. Mandy, now 60 years old, had first been diagnosed with MS at the age of 23. She had produced four children all of whom took great pride in looking after her and making what was left of her life as tolerable as possible. Every day she would go to the gym to fight her illness and keep it as far at bay as she possibly could. It was a titanic battle. The MS was resolutely trying to retain its stranglehold on her disposition every bit as much as she was determined to prevent it from taking her life over completely. She formed a tepee in her walking style as, using two sticks she spread her legs out straight at forty-five degrees behind and apart while plonking the sticks at a similar jaunt ahead. Going for a stroll was a thing of her distant past, getting across a room was now a military campaign. You could see the torture etched across her face as she sat upon the rowing machine and had her hands wrapped in Velcro so that she could grip the handlebars which pulled the weights to enable her shoulders to flex and stretch.

She was a real fighter; someone who never ever moaned about her lot and the most stunning example of strength in adversity.

The centre has been relocated now as the building has been knocked down to make way for luxury apartments. A new facility has been created in a smartly furbished purpose-built Queen Mary's hospital thanks to the Labour Party's determination to spend vast amounts of money on bigger corridors for all.

I have never felt so utterly detached from my general practitioner as I do in today's society and am determined that if I ever have anything again which I think might be mildly serious I would go straight to accident and emergencies. If the police forces move their offices there too perhaps I could buy my petrol, have my fingerprints checked, leave a blood sample and collect my weekly groceries at the same time.

Certainly we needed to overhaul the outdated and perfunctory collection of hospital buildings across our land. Yet did we intend, in all conscience, to imbalance the relationship between preventative medicine and care last provided by community doctors a generation ago by so openly encouraging people to go straight to hospital? My own experience teaches me that unless I want a placebo or to waste time with my GP who is only going to refer me to a specialist anyway, I might just as well admit myself directly. Your average GP is a bright bloke, armed with years of training and knowledge. He, like many thoroughbred creatures, needs exercise, particularly for his brain.

Friends and relations continued to come and visit. They still had to negotiate around my times of physiotherapy which totalled about twenty hours a week. It was so much nicer to be able to welcome people into your own environment and to allow their health of body and mind to encourage, infect and nurture you.

Cousins and friends had travelled from as far away as America and Hong Kong. One had given me a DVD entitled The Motorcycle Diaries. It is a story of an idealistic, educated, charismatic and handsome young man who postpones his training to become a doctor in order to set off on a journey of discovery that would take him on a tour of South America setting off from Buenos Aires, his hometown, across Argentina to Chile up to Peru taking in Paraguay and Venezuela. He ends up doing voluntary work in a leper colony and never goes home.

His idealism takes such a hold of his life that any craven thoughts are banished and with great bravery he then sets off to work with guerrillas in Cuba.

His name was Che Guevara who swapped the roistering good time he had sampled while exploring the Andes for a life of attrition prematurely terminated.

There was plenty of piety and poetry in this film but its raw beauty lay in the exploration of his continent with his best friend and their battle with nature, lack of money, and the vagaries of a Triumph 250 Bonneville's engine.

It should be essential viewing for anyone who has suffered an illness.

On the chart of 'there is always someone worse off than you', where do you think suffering from leprosy sits? In Crete they used to give the lepers their own island but took away their liberty and self-respect. Don't sneer though because you never wasted a moment before pondering whether to give up the Isle of Skye or perhaps Hayling Island if you were faced with the equivalent dilemma; or for that matter where to deposit a leper's self-respect or quarantine their liberty.

At this stage of the illness I still can't tie my own shoelaces properly or undo the buttons on my shirt in less than twenty minutes. I can lift my arms in the air and give an approximate impression of a normal person shaking hands. The only difference appears to be 'Are you in the Masons?' , a question I am invariably asked when disengaging hands as my index finger curls around in on itself, getting squashed in the shake process. This is compounded by my inability to retrieve my hand, as my thumb also gets in on the act by wrapping itself around the back of the hand of any poor innocent soul unfortunate enough to have to do the handshake dance with me.

To correct this and my other malfunctions I flex my finger and hand muscles to wake them from their torpor whenever I can. It's a great way to pass the time on journeys. Like when we set off in a sensory bus, so called because it makes a beeping sound when reversing towards cars, walls and other objects. I had hoped for something more winsome when first espying the legend 'sensory' on the side of the bus. A melange of aromatherapy oils, joss sticks, music by Enya, some scented candles with rose petal water and so on, might have made our journey over the South Circular Road more of an experience.

We touch our forelocks to the daily sight of a shrine to the much lamented, died too young, driving his mini motor car too fast, lived life to the full, under the influence of hallucinagenics whilst riding the White Swan, Marc Bolan. Pictures of him in his King Charles 1st wig, in full make-up with star dust sprinkled in his heavily tressed locks still adorn two trees near Barnes railway station, in a display of such glittering tackiness that even a magpie would be ashamed.

Is it better to die young?

How much less idealised would our opinions be of Marc Bolan or Princess Diana if they had turned 50, suffered a stroke, lost the use of one side of their body and the ability and will to speak? These thoughts ride with me on the way to the Douglas Bader gym in Roehampton; our special-purpose facility for the disabled and those who have lost limbs.

The numbers had been greatly enhanced when the London bombing incidents of the Seventh of July had gone off.

People going about their business in all innocence; Completely oblivious to the mortal threat that existed within rucksacks and holdalls attached to some very dim British-born young men determined to martyr themselves in what was to them a very noble cause. The resultant carnage made the headlines of newspapers around the world, the effect though could be measured in the faces and empty stares of the victims trying to rebuild their shattered lives at this very gymnasium.

The thought that suspected terrorists should be locked up for 90 days without trial was top of the debating agenda for weeks, and I read the pro's and con's with interest. For all the hot air expended it should not have been possible to determine a wholesale change in our constitution without seeing at first hand the results of these young men's actions.

To have your legs blown off, lose an eye and your best friend and still retain your love of all mankind was a big ask.

No sooner had I disembarked from the sensory bus and entered the building, than a young woman in her early thirties on crutches with two new metal legs attached from the thigh downwards strode past me giggling. She was wearing shorts which exposed the pipe work, ducting and intricacies of the metal limbs that had been added to her new body. Complete with a pair of trainers wrapped around her false feet she might have been excused a moment of despondency. Yet there she was in a state of high excitement roaring with laughter as a lugubrious technician came along behind her holding a can of oil in his left hand and a large screwdriver in his right, exclaiming, 'I think your right leg is moving a bit slow, sit down for goodness sake!' She had no reason to bless the seventh of July and every excuse to curse it, but she was damned if she was going to stop enjoying her life.

This scene contrasted wildly with the upsurge in events which were beginning to put me back into mainstream activities. I was trying to split my week from a disabled one on Mondays, Wednesdays and Fridays to an able bodied time on Tuesdays and Thursdays. So it was on the first Tuesday of the month that we ventured out to eat. This in preparation for the much bigger and real challenge of going back to work.

My favourite restaurant in England is called Bibendum which is housed in the old Michelin building on the first floor.

Although lovely at night I prefer it at lunchtime because it has stained glass windows to encourage the sunshine to beam its dappled light across the high ceiling. Violets, indigos, petrol blues, emerald apples and chiffon yellows dance on your tablecloth and glassware.

The tables are never set too close together and the food is always sharp, simple, well observed and bloody good. The service can be a bit French at times, you know stuffy, supercilious and a bit up itself but on the whole I just like the space. Many people think of it as Terence Conran's first restaurant. Strictly this is not true because he designed the now defunct Harveys restaurant in the wine cellars of Denmark Street in Bristol in the 1960s.

Cellars which I got to know rather well with its fine collection of Nailsea Blue and Red glass which would dominate my thoughts many years later when I launched an indigo blue mineral water bottle on an unsuspecting world three months before Perrier had their Benzene scare.

This outing was to mark a late birthday acknowledgement because I had not been strong enough to venture out on the day itself so soon after leaving the rehabilitation centre. Two great friends joined us and the occasion went swimmingly; that was until we got to the point at the end of the meal when I needed to go to the loo. We had made the mistake of selecting a pair of proper trousers, which had a zip on the front, a belt and buckle. Rank bad planning on my part, I confess. There wasn't a disabled toilet on the same floor and Suzi felt uncomfortable taking me into the gents.

We excused ourselves to all the ladies present in their loo on our way in as though this was a perfectly normal routine for a disabled man on sticks like some postprandial ritual. Getting into the narrow cubicle was difficult enough but the hard part was doing my trousers up again when I had finished, I couldn't do this myself. I hissed instructions trying to keep my voice low while Suzi squatted down to get my fly at her eye level. You might be thinking that this was starting to look a bit saucy.

Parallels perhaps with Boris Becker having all the fun turning a broom cupboard at the Metropolitan hotel into the most frequently asked for space in the building and accordingly the most expensive British letting space in cost per square inch/foot/divorce?

I was desperately trying to think about anything else but inches that might be squaring up as the cubicle was barged open by an intemperate harridan who exclaimed 'Disgusting! On what possible basis can you justify such salacious behaviour, get out now before I report you to the authorities!' I confess that at that very moment Suzi's hand was stuck inside my zip and her mouth was wide open in horror as this officer of the toilet police vented her spleen.

On reflection the evidence did not look too good. I was smiling with sapient pleasure having enjoyed an epicurean feast in the dining room and Suzi was licking her lips because she always sticks out her tongue whenever she is concentrating (honest!). If we had been able to leave with our tails firmly between our legs than that is how we would have departed. Instead we rose above the kafuffle and left the ladies' loo with our heads held high, delighting in matching the verbal assault with a suitably pithy riposte 'Thank you so much for introducing yourself, the pleasure was all ours!' Ever since I have planned my choice of the right trousers as studiously as the route to any gourmet tour.

On an able-bodied Thursday I went to a friend's house for an alfresco supper by the river. I first met Martin on a boys golfing trip to the Caribbean. We played a round together on the first day and he forgot the sun cream. He tried to see the funny side when the rest of the guys all ordered lobster for breakfast the following day. Wearing a long sleeved shirt, two gloves and a wide brimmed hat he gamely tried to play again while his arms, nose and neck turned an even brighter pink. We kept in touch regularly over the years thereafter until Martin announced that he was going to collect me from the hospital and take me to his house for dinner.

The chauffeur arrived in an anthracite grey Bentley upon which I now consider myself to be an expert. The Bentley Mulsane Turbo is without doubt a great car. It is great because the boot will take a Zimmer frame in one go and a wheelchair at the same time. The doors are so wide you can swing your legs in and better still adjust the seat height.

Next time you see one go past and think to yourself 'flash bastard' or even worse 'footballer' just remember that in my fantasy society if I get my way they will be standard issue to all people with disabilities while the rest of the time able-bodied folk will have to cram themselves into a mini or 2CV.

The meal by the river was a triumph of ambition over logic as I couldn't get down the pathway without being carried/lifted/pushed, but my trousers held firm. Martin meanwhile, as well as being a Shintu priest, travel agent and bundle of frenetic energy was turning his attentions to Albania and in particular its forgotten vineyards. A much more interesting topic than Polish plumbers for our cappuccino classes to debate, don't you think? What about "how is your erectile function", closely followed by "I was talking to my Albanian viniculturist the other day" to kick off your next pretentious dinner party?

Mark you, staying with the priapic theme, I did read that Durham had been described as a 'lambent willy' the other day. And that does take the pretentious biscuit. Although it might be a good name for a pop group, but then so might 'pretentious biscuit'.

If laughing at myself, laced with rants against disabled body prejudices, had provided part of the mental recovery recipe, then relentless physiotherapy had been my guiding body bible. Mondays had become the local work out morning, going to a gym half a mile from the house and placing my welfare in the hands of Paul, a cheerful uber-fit young man of east London origin who for the last ten years had specialised in guiding disabled folks like me by freelancing from gym to gym on his pushbike. He must have helped over 200 people in a week darting from one venue to the next class, but he knew exactly how to make me feel that I was the most important man in the world. He was absolutely the sort of bloke that should receive an MBE commendation for unsung hero activities.

Monday afternoons, though, were for work! Yes it was time to get the brain back into gear and see if I could add any value to the directors I had so inconsiderately dropped in it all those eons ago. A couple of hours a week may seem laughable but it was a start and it allowed me a peek at the problems women experience when they depart their work desk to have babies and leave all their confidence behind in the in tray.

Before this moment I had in my male blinkered stupidity assumed that work was like riding a horse, if you fell off then you got straight back on.

Poppycock, you also leave your knowledge, contacts, pace, brio, importance and relevance behind. Assuming a role of importance again would require patience and indulgence from my work colleagues. I would also need their permission but picking up the threads of what was relevant was much scarier. How dare I? How could I possibly offer relevant advice let alone instruction when I had been in another universe for so long?

That was the crux of my 'how to get on with work mates' dilemma.

How to master the client challenge would take new bravery pills and lots of trial and error.

Physically my present status quo simply wasn't enough anymore. I was becoming increasingly impatient with daily exercise to stimulate the nerve endings. I was ready to try something more exotic. Work rations for starters and alternate medical devices for main course.

Eleven months after first collapsing I met up with Dr Roberto Ciaff, which is not Italian for Chav. For 25 years he had been combining his qualifications in medicine with a fascination for electronic engineering.

Initially targeting the Motor Neurone patient he had perfected a method which sent electronic impulses through the body to enhance the pace of regeneration in the nervous system. The early exchanges did not fill me with supreme confidence. I was invited to put my feet into a bucket of water and was then linked up to the national grid as a variety of electric impulses were projected into me. The process was then repeated on my hands. Miraculously the pain in my fingers abated, not forever, but just enough to remind me what it felt like to have something approaching normal sensation restored.

From doubting Thomas to disciple in an instant; I have been back countless times making my weekly pilgrimage to Oxted. We have progressed from bucket immersion to direct application of pads to the spine, thighs and elbows with a variety of positive and negative pulses coursing through my veins. Plus and minus, left and right boogie, marching up the hill and the tumble dryer represent the code names for the base components of my electric workout. With this machinery I'm able to take my legs on a route march over a far greater distance than if I tried to walk. There is no cardiovascular involvement but it is surprising to feel the effect that an electric impulse targeted, say, on the knee has on the shoulder.

The principles of acupuncture still apply but the best analogy I can think of to describe the effect lies in the image of a foot pressed firmly down over a hosepipe with the tap turned on full blast. That is how the body feels in the hibernating parts before the electric impulse treatment sets about its work. Drilling away at blockages until key nerves wake up, the foot is lifted off the pipe, and the body of energy and power which has built up behind the dam is set free.

At the beginning most settings were turned to maximum to get as much juice through my system as possible to clear the debris. Now I'm only able to tolerate relatively small doses because areas of sensitivity have been rediscovered. Target areas enlarge because the motorways that carry the messages from brain to target and back again have been cleared by highway patrol.

By happenstance I missed a few weeks before completing this story and did not realise how addicted I had become to the process and the resultant buzz. The system works by at least providing temporary relief and will, I suspect, become standard procedure for application on people with wasting illnesses like MS, as the wider medical profession comes to accept the process.

It is already second nature to senior sports teams whose carefully tuned and thoroughbred athletic torsos require the finest of fine tuning. It is not just steroids and muscle bulking agents for our professional sportsmen these days.

The electric workout is here to stay. But was I here to stay or was some sort of ending in sight? Christmas was fast approaching, anniversary time. A time to give enormous thanks that I'm still here, much improved by comparison with this time last year. I have got most of the Christmas cards ready to post, the presents are allocated and wrapped, and as the shortest day of the year, the 21st, breaks at dawn I proffer a little prayer to all my gods for their forbearance.

For 12 months now I have been sidelined to the emergency pit stop whilst the rest of the world raced by.

Can you please stop the world? I want to get back on!

Not possible yet, I'm afraid. I can only manage to undo shoelaces but can't do them up. I can put food into my mouth with a spoon but can't cut it with a knife. I can undo some buttons on my shirt but can't get my left arm into the sleeve or do any buttons up. The list goes on, something and nothing, so near and so far.

Parts of my body almost look normal from the outside. The hands and feet receive messages intermittently offering pain and imprecision as their excuse for not writing home. My trunk, back and sides I assume are reasonably normal because they don't hurt as much, yet even they are not tuned into the right frequency. The fertile bits that are growing back to the previous reality are matched by equal patches of wasteland that remain barren in terms of response.

A year is a long time. Quite long enough to document this story before I lose your attention. My patience is wearing thinner, as I get closer to being able to do something correctly, so my temper shortens. The time when I had no choice but to abdicate sovereignty over my frame is long past.

Tantalisingly faculties are returning in random order.

It is supremely frustrating trying to allot independent action back to functions like walking and writing because neither of them is roadworthy enough to pass their MOT.

Meanwhile Sundance is at home in sheltered accommodation confined to bed, some days, able to walk freely on others, inspired by his children and looking for romance in Whitby where he has met a fellow MS sufferer who is rather sweet on him. They are busy perfecting 'the love maker's guide to romance in wheelchairs' which is sure to be a bestseller and before you ask, it is best to use at least two chairs in the process.

The crew at the hospital in Bath are much the same except for the introduction of a new matron who is busy dishing out the orders, same as the old matron. Plus ça change... Kirsten has become a stalker! Having followed her boyfriend's change of jobs she has moved to London and just knocked at my door to begin our next physio session. She has taken over the local outpatient supervision programme and to our joint surprise has been awarded me as her first case. She is the most welcome sight and tears of unbounded pleasure cascade down my snivelling face.

Her arrival brings vivid memories flooding back of how Suzi and I celebrated the first six months of recovery by leaving the hospital for an excellent afternoon's adventure in a 'taxi'.

It was a small minibus with an electrically controlled ramp which enabled wheelchairs to be pushed up and inside in one movement and afforded me my first chance to explore the world beyond the hospital campus. Kirsten had suggested it as we had been invited out to tea by a beautiful/handsome woman called Lisa. Thirty-two years previously she had owned a restaurant near Bath and had the great misfortune to employ me as an ancillary waiter. I hadn't seen her for years but curiously had accused one of the junior doctors in the intensive care department of being her daughter so striking was the resemblance. She was also called Lisa.

The serendipity of life took a further turn when who should I spy turning the corridor two weeks later on her way to visit another patient than the original Lisa.

It was her idea that we should visit her house in a taxi and she took care of all the arrangements. Her home is the most stunning 16th century property in a hidden valley just outside Bath offering a perfect blend of solitude and proximity. Access was hopeless for a wheelchair so her partner Donald heaved me in through the front door.

The quintessential English summer's day demonstrated perfectly why we always talk about the weather. The sun came out to play sporadically amidst dark clouds interrupted by a magnificent rainbow with all seven colours gleaming in their Harlequin glory while the logs on the fire crackled, spat and smoked and we sipped Earl Grey tea, mine through a straw, and savoured the freshest cucumber sandwiches.

The man who Lisa had been visiting in hospital was an immediate neighbour of hers in the valley. Christopher in his early Sixties had been struck down by a stroke in his left side just before one of his daughters was due to give birth to his first grandchild and the other was about to get married. So determined was he to walk his daughter down the aisle and attend the birth that Christopher overdosed on physiotherapy.

Never mind his neuralgia, or the moments when he fell over, he was competition! Until then I thought I was the one showing the most cussed determination. Valentine, his redoubtable and charming wife, had no idea what an inspiration her husband was to me to double my efforts.

Meanwhile she lent me cassette tapes ranging from a bit of Le Carre to Samuel Pepys diaries, doubling the rations of food for the brain indeed!

Rations of love were an entirely different matter as I had been so poor at handing any out. I remember how long it had taken my youngest son to come to terms with the fact that I was so unwell. It was at the six month turning point when he had asked me as he was about to leave the bedside one sultry afternoon.

'How do you clean your teeth, Dad?' I replied, 'Someone does it for me.' He nodded and then asked, 'and how do you put your clothes on?' I repeated, 'Someone does it for me.'

It was as though a penny was finally dropping. For all the love that he had offered unconditionally had been based on a suspension of reality. Dad is supposed to be there to rely upon, to be solid and dependable and I wasn't doing a very good job of convincing him of my strength or durability.

A six month sojourn had turned into twelve, missing out on watching him grow up entering his 18th year, wrestling with his A-levels and his choice of further education. Time that I could never get back or reverse. But there is never a good time to be ill, it just comes along and punches you on the nose when you least expect. His original artwork for which he claimed the school's golden paintbrush award, no less, is the cover of this book. "Faces of Confinement" lives on. It was his way of showing support. He found it easier to talk to his art master about my health than he did to my face, a sentiment which I totally understand. Not to be outdone by Charlie, my eldest son Sam bashed out a few records to an innocent 'my space' public and selected one track to sit on the www.ghee-yan-bah-ray.com website, which he built to help me and others get by. It's called 'Heart' and he is full of it. In her own way George was as supportive and helpful as I had any right to expect let alone hope for and performed so many acts of mercy and assistance behind the scenes that if I said thank you for each one it would take me till tomorrow.

For today was becoming far less important and tomorrow would only belong to me if I could just shake off the mindset. Discarding it and moving on from being ill to establishing a new well regime needs more than an attitude of mind, though. You need advice and others' past experience to lean on.

Charles de la Main at the age of 22 was in the mood for celebration. He charged headlong into a swimming pool with glee which abruptly turned to horror as he hit the surface and realised how shallow the water was. His back broke in the process. He spent the next eight months in a state of abject surrender cocooned inside a plaster cast which prevented him from moving his torso at all. This did not stop him from making a full recovery and continuing to career through life like the cavalier he was born to be. When Charles spoke I listened intently because he was one of the few visitors who had shared the experience of long term debilitation. His speech was considered and precise as he proceeded to debunk the assumptions that I had made about recovery.

When you are better and people say 'How are you?', just say, 'Fine thank you.' You will want to explain every last detail of your experience and won't see how quickly people's eyes glaze over. You will not be box office news for any length of time, believe me, people just won't want to know.

My quandary was to determine at what time to announce to the world that I was on the way back.

So I set an arbitrary point exactly one year after my admission to the first hospital reasoning that by announcing that I was better a level of self-fulfilment would kick in the more I repeated the phrase.

Granted I still need a lot of help from Kenneth the kindly care worker who wakes me each morning and enables me to take increasing levels of responsibility for my own ablutions. Agreed I can't use my hands properly to dial a telephone number or write an almanac of the last year. You are right to observe that I still am not able to dress myself, handle loose change or make a hot drink independently. The authorities won't allow me to drive and my paperwork confirms that I am disabled.

Even though my body has been ameliorating along at a slower pace than my mindset and in truth there are many years of relentless physiotherapy activity to go, I'm not prepared to wait any longer.

This story needs to have a happy ending and society will just have to ignore the lack of sartorial elegance, my gait which resembles the Tin Man from the Wizard of Oz and my sporadic lack of zest. I have started to learn to play bridge and although I can't deal, shuffle or even hold my cards, it does not stop me playing. When I first arrived at the card school I could see the other novices staring at me in trepidation as I inched towards them on my walking frame. Cupping their hands across their mouths and whispering to their immediate neighbour, 'Please don't let the freak sit next to me.' There was a time when this would have made me timorous but not any more.

This is the point where I want to stop being classed as off sick. It may only be a psychological sleight of hand or mind but it's enough.

This chronicle has to stop. I am recovered enough to consign my 50th year to its own resting place.

From hereon in I want to be treated as a well person. So please don't ask me any more questions because the answer you will get is 'Just fine, thank you.'

Then my dad died.

"Needs re-reading and re-visiting several times over to let it all sink in" - Clive Mantle, Actor ('Casualty' Dr Mike Barrett)

*** *** ***

"An incredible journey and a privilege to read" - Dr. Martin Godfrey, past Editor 'Pulse'

*** *** ***

"Well, frankly I'm disappointed. I had expected it to be mostly about us and how much our existence mattered to the author, and that it needed GBS to teach him this simple but obvious truth. But he redeemed himself with a delicious Freudian slip about staying 'intact' with the bloke who hired the axe murderers!" - Patrick and Ivo Tennant, 'The Daily Telegraph'

CHAPTER NINE
ASHES TO ANGER

The utter futility and sense of loss should have been easy to predict and plan for but I felt overwhelmed, destitute, trapped and very, very angry..

There were many reasons for the breadth of change in my mood. Let me explain.

When you leave a restaurant on a winter's night, put on your overcoat and step out into the chill air, think of me. Don't get too cross, though.

I admit I made a mistake when I left wearing your real coat five minutes earlier. You won't ever know who I am but you will struggle to smile as the realisation dawns on you that your much loved coat either doesn't fit anymore or won't be coming back. The coat over your shoulders looked oh so familiar... while in a parallel universe I am struggling to work out why what I thought was my coat doesn't fit. The difference is that I can't swap it or buy a new one. Every day I wake up and put someone else's coat over my body, every day it feels like it belongs to some other being and every day the battle is lost to get my frame to fit itself. Yes it bloody well hurts but worse, it makes me so angry.

It is a long time since I left the Wolfson thinking I could smell the air as I made my last escape. Saying good bye to the retired army officer and musing over the things that most concerned us about being pushed out of the hospital and back into the community; such as when the kindly general asked me the killer question in his clipped military tone, 'Do you mind if I ask you a very, very personal question?'… 'No, of course not please go ahead'… 'Well it's a bit awkward but it troubles me so'… 'No really it's fine'… 'Can you wipe your own arse?'…. 'No, I can't'…. 'Oh good… neither can I.'

Learning to ablute yourself takes patience, practice and perseverance…it is best not to do it in some other person's overcoat. I'm not bad at it now, not good on an international, competitive level, just not bad. In itself this doesn't make me that angry.

I wish I could say the same for my nose wiping because that should be really excellent but no matter what I try I can't really smell the air. I can't smell anything properly. No lavender in Provence, scented lemons from Sicily, or freshly baked bread.

No Chanel 'No.5', no rose petals, hyacinths or Gatling's farts. All smells are history, absented from the rest of the senses perhaps to return… perhaps not.

Which would you choose to lose, sight, hearing, taste?

These all seem relatively intact but touch and smell have been distant friends for a long time. Yes touch is changing, as I get infinitesimal shifts in my personal paradigm when tiny extra shards of feeling return to my toes and fingers. That is when the GBS Stasi deem it appropriate to amortise my loss. Now a lack of smell is inconvenient and a nuisance but the combined lack of smell and touch are frustrating and entrapping.

So I try to believe that if you are able to keep your sight, hearing, taste, and most crucially your peripheral vision or sixth sense intact you are still doing relatively okay.

I can see beans on toast. It's easy to picture cinnamon sticks in mulled wine, or remember the malt shroud that sat so thick and square over Waverley station in Edinburgh but how they smell now I have no idea. Perhaps it will come back in a return to sender packet with the parcels man from the post office thumping at my door. Maybe there is just one pong that holds the key to unlock my nasal passages and once it has found the magic pathway an avalanche of whiffs and sniffs, odours, scents and fragrances will re-awaken the redundant passages in my mind.

I would probably choose to lose smell too, same as you. Especially now I've got anger in my belly to keep me company, after all that calm acceptance of my lot has evaporated.

There are subtleties with the other senses though, so for instance my hearing is relatively intact but my heart is older now, much older, and this gives me the excuse to behave without recourse to my actual age or hearing.

'Have you any butter?' I bellow at the old man running the nearest convenience shop, taking up my new self-styled status as a 72 year old, who's left his ear trumpet at home.

'Turn down that fearful racket on your radio, cabbie!' I boom away in my senior contempt, oblivious to the sensibilities of those who have entered this removed world in which I now reside. A world in which you scratch along, hoping for stimulation and succour.

They say heroin years are lost. That those who become addicted suspend normality and never get those wilderness times back. I imagine this is similar because the precociousness of my youth has long been abandoned; the optimism of middle age bypassed and the fast forward button has projected me way beyond my actual age. Although I am trying to turn the clock back, the evidence is clear. I am going to be trapped here as a grumpy old man, if I don't put up a fight.

But this is not vital, merely a side show, by comparison with a man's needs.

Arousal is a combination of so many senses that one going missing is bound to piss off the others. There was a time when my whole torso could feel aroused in a trice but the knit of bodily stimuli so complete hitherto has stopped working and I can no longer tell if I am coming or going. For girls the erogenous zones can be very precise but for us fellas your back, your stomach, even your arms get involved... turning the utilitarian nature of the body's job into something far more esoteric. Or at least I think that is how it used to be.

Sex is a motivating force, often blind in its indeterminate path but for me it has been emasculated off the agenda to make a welcome but occasional guest appearance. The body's force field is on safari, no more an erogenous zone than an erroneous one. Would this make you angry?

I will get over these things. Like all the barriers surmounted previously they are there to be scaled, broken, removed or torn down. Restoring interest in bodily pleasure will be easy one day but getting over my dad's death put all thoughts of 'I'm fine, thank you' down the proverbial toilet.

This Tsunami was from a different ocean but like the Atlantic storm that first hit me it turned nasty and the world I had tried so hard to rebuild came crashing down all over again. The futility of all my efforts trying to put life back onto an even keel, were laid bare for open inspection.

A big black hole engulfed me and I dived down into the very depths of myopic despond. Why now? Couldn't you just let me be a bit stronger to get back to caring for him? How can I be expected to write an obituary, organise a funeral, invite all his friends and relations, book the wake and do those bastard shoelaces up?

I don't want to be trapped here in an alien body when I so desperately need all my faculties back. I don't need jocular asides to cheer me up like, "They say old professors never die they just lose their faculties". Because I guess they feel trapped too but by stipend and campus and have less need of the anger management course running through my head.

The solitary confinement was under renewed assault. Yes, my body most certainly had been attacked but my mind had not given in, until now. I was so bleedingly, contemptuously, splenetically, and profoundly angry because, buried as it had been, dad's death finally made the suppressed boils of emotional bile and contempt erupt, exploding like the most brutal volcano.

For all my self-pity and protestations it was a calm mind which had learnt how to reconnect with all the love that I mistakenly thought had disappeared into cold storage in the freezer outside. It had taken time and great patience but it was now shaken to the core. The love of life and giving to others had taken time to filter through. Drawn perhaps by osmosis or morphed by Mr. Spock. Back in wave after wave from the rose garden to which I assumed it had been banished all those months ago, and now this.

It was a big loss.

The loss of any unconditional love is always a shock because to receive it in the first place is such a bonus in life and certainly not our birthright.

The sadness of his passing made me feel worse for sure, down and down went the mood, blacker and blacker went the sky but as the storm clouds broke, so a freshness emerged. The anger began slowly to subside.

A certainty that he would always be at my side washed over me in tandem with, but outweighing the waves of melancholy. Before I knew it a decision was made in my subconscious; to finally stop writing this book and feeling so selfishly sorry for myself and look forward with new purpose. It was, and still is, that 'giving' of strength to others from my father which took the lid off my coffin.

Even though the responsibility curve had swung its full arc years before and I had been his carer for ages, this last passage had made us brothers in our infirm arms. This was an equalisation; a certainty of knowledge had arrived to confirm that I could now mimic his mannerisms with impunity. They had been genetically absorbed, but I had fought so hard to subconsciously deny the inheritance. At last this self-deception was no longer necessary, the trap was broken.

I had known it was there, all right, but somehow it had seemed so tantalising out of reach…

Dad was a big man, 6'8 in his prime, yet a gentle, gentleman in all his manners.

He literally ran out of breath at the end, having been in and out of hospital for most of the year since his 90th. On Thursday in his last week, he was definitely rallying but on the Friday his breathing dipped alarmingly and he was ambulanced to the A and E department of the Bristol Royal Infirmary. They kept him alive until we, his family, could get there but the sepsis was so overwhelming that he couldn't keep breathing unsupported.

So, surrounded by his loved ones, we held his hand, told him we would always be with him and watched him literally run out of puff and slip away.

He had become terribly hot, so a fan had been placed close to him to rotate across his face. His white hair was sticking out wafting upwards in the breeze.

It kept moving after he had left us, still trying to make us smile with his unwitting Mr Pastry impersonation.

I am sure he continues to laugh and smile upon us even now.

He gave me my moral compass, which I fought to observe, over 50 years of that unconditional love and a fund of stories, jokes, asides and observations that I will never forget. He witnessed two world wars, the Suez crisis, the Falkland war, the invasion of Iraq, the birth of motor cars, television and the Internet, while sticking blissfully to his golden era in which the omnipotent Bing Crosby ruled the air waves.

Towards the end he needed more help with daily chores than a man of his pride wanted to allow. He was the best Dad and friend I could have hoped for.

He was a compassionate man. Learn from his lesson. Put the anger back in its box.

On the Monday after my dad died in Bristol there was an operation back in south London. That meant returning to the hospital, where they had sewn my head together after a fall. I wasn't looking forward to it; but nothing prepared me for the sight of three fully armed policemen in flak jackets brandishing semi-automatic weapons next to the waiting room in which I waited for the surgeons to correct another of my impediments.

There had been, 'a Shootin' in Tootin' which had taken place that morning outside the doors of the hospital and they feared reprisals... it did not help elevate my sense of inner calm or 'sphincter' control. As this was the part of me about to be reduced to one from its greedy dual status. Any hint of anger here would have been quoshed instantly, so I cheered myself up by attributing a new line to my ridiculous hero. As Ricky Tomlinson would have said so Roylely, 'security, my arse!'

I needed a day to recover from the anaesthetic, tentatively perching on lots of comfy cushions before we could get down to the very serious business of organizing a fitting tribute. We had the funeral service a few days later and thoughts of crying were absented. The day was a triumph of organisation and cooperation from all our friends and helpers. It passed into history as it does for all families and the tears of sadness, joy and relief came, thankfully, when everyone had gone home.

Suzi did everything in her power to lift me out of the abyss and we have much to be grateful for but while the trap today is slightly less restricting, it's still there. The prison service without bars and the sense of 'a solitary confinement' remain my companions.

Other illnesses may come and go but few pervade like GBS with its limpet-like desire to stick around. It has made me invisible to many, it's made people stare straight through me or ignore me; A reflection of my self-regard perhaps, but an ignominy unplanned for sure.

It has imposed huge restrictions on others and permanently diverted the course of their lives. It's removed my sense of smell and touch, triggered problems with my walking, removed my independence, devastated my sex drive and energy levels, taken away years of my life, introduced relentless physiotherapy, made me totally reconsider how to explain myself in business, given me untold pain as my one abiding constant, removed me from my children, changed forever my dress code, transformed the way I see others' boorish behaviour and even stopped my body and mind from being joined up.

It has been one hell of an epiphany.

But I am going to beat it, no matter how long it takes.

Lest you think me always sad though, let me leave you with a smile.

Picture the changes needed in the frequency and nature of going on holiday which have now been forced upon us. That I can even take a holiday makes me a lucky man. A holiday from what, you might ask? Well I have gotten back into the work saddle, given myself permission to take charge and worked out how to behave in sufficiently normal a way in business that I can safely say I'm back. On conditional discharge perhaps, but definitely back.

When Suzi and I get on a plane we use a wheelchair. It's too far for me to walk from public transport to the airport terminal and I try not to let my pride get in the way of practicality. The man assigned to get us on board is fast approaching and guess what?

He has only got one arm. But remember, it's the only one that works properly between us!

I thought about saying something sympathetic but it didn't come out that way. I recalled how those children in the park at Wimbledon would have reacted and then it just pops out; A sentence under new public ownership.

'I don't want to go around in circles,' I jest.

At first there is silence, then very, very slowly.........He begins to laugh,

We laugh,

The couple next to us start to laugh, then the whole queue behind us laughs.

As the entire departure lounge sniggers aloud to this hopelessly incorrect thing to say, we are served a reminder. It is like life itself. Cruel at times for sure, but the 'always someone worse off than you are' school of philosophy is so bitingly accurate. You have to accept the doctrine and give thanks for the blessings you do have, no matter how small they may be. Before that bell tolls.

No one said life was easy, but determination, persistence, anger harnessed in the right way and above all patience will take you such a long way.

After all, doesn't GBS stand for Getting Better Slowly?

The End

All proceeds from the sale of this book will be given to the GBS society to help fight the illness and raise funds for further research.

Printed in the United Kingdom
by Lightning Source UK Ltd.
126784UK00001B/124-135/A